Waste Knot: Creative Cooking Techniques for a Greener Family Kitchen

MONICA LYNNE CHASE

In Waste Knot: Creative Cooking Techniques for a Greener Family Kitchen, Monica Lynne Chase invites readers to reimagine their kitchen as a space for sustainability and creativity. This book offers practical techniques to minimize food waste, repurpose leftovers, and make the most of every ingredient. From root-to-stem recipes to innovative meal planning strategies, it empowers families to embrace eco-conscious habits without sacrificing flavor or nutrition. With a focus on plant-based and grain-free options, Waste Knot serves as a guide for those looking to reduce their environmental impact, save money, and create delicious, wholesome meals that benefit both their family and the planet.

Table of Contents:

Chapter 1: introduction to sustainable cooking
Chapter 2: plant-based meal prep
Chapter 3: locally sourced super foods
Chapter 4: eco-friendly packaging solutions
Chapter 5: nutrient dense smoothie recipes
Chapter 6: low waist, cooking techniques
Chapter 7: herbal and medicinal foods
Chapter 8: family, friendly, sustainable recipes
Chapter 9: engaging teen cooks in sustainable practices
Chapter 10: building a sustainable kitchen culture

Recipes:

1. **Root to stem veggie stir-fry**
2. **Leftover lentil shepherds pie**
3. **Zero waste vegetable broth**
4. **Carrot top pesto**

References & Resources

Chapter One: Introduction to Sustainable Cooking

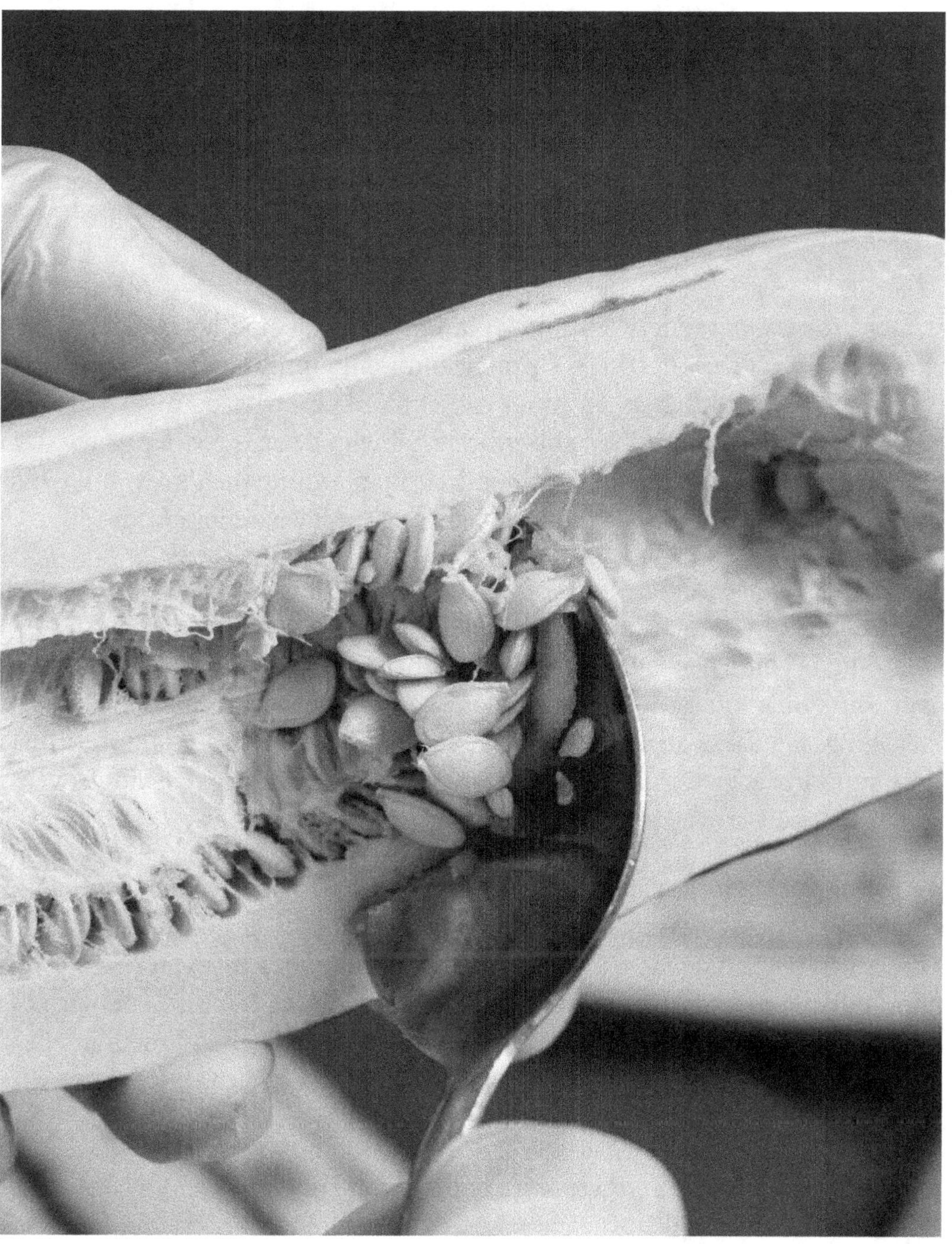

The Importance of Waste Reduction

Waste reduction is a crucial practice for families looking to adopt a more sustainable lifestyle in the kitchen. By minimizing waste, families not only contribute to environmental preservation but also enhance their health and wellness. Each year, a staggering amount of food is discarded, leading to increased greenhouse gas emissions and unnecessary strain on landfills. By prioritizing waste reduction, families can actively participate in combating climate change while enjoying the benefits of fresher, healthier meals.

One effective strategy for waste reduction is meal planning, which enables cooks to purchase only the ingredients they need. This practice not only minimizes food waste but also fosters creativity in the kitchen. Families can explore plant-based meal prep by incorporating seasonal and locally sourced superfoods, which not only reduce waste but also support local farmers and promote a healthier diet. By planning meals around what is in season, families can create nutrient-dense dishes that are both delicious and environmentally friendly.

Another important aspect of waste reduction is the use of eco-friendly packaging solutions. Many products come packaged in materials that contribute to pollution and waste. By choosing bulk bins, reusable containers, and products with minimal or compostable packaging, families can significantly reduce their environmental footprint. This shift not only supports a sustainable lifestyle but can also lead to cost savings over time, as buying in bulk often proves to be more economical.

In addition to reducing packaging waste, families can also focus on low-waste cooking techniques that make the most of every ingredient. Utilizing vegetable scraps, stems, and peels can transform potential waste into flavorful stocks, sauces, or even snacks. This approach not only maximizes the use of purchased ingredients but also encourages mindfulness about food consumption. Moreover, incorporating herbal and medicinal foods into recipes can enhance nutritional value while promoting health, further emphasizing the importance of using every part of the food.

Ultimately, the importance of waste reduction extends beyond environmental concerns. It fosters a culture of creativity, health consciousness, and sustainability within families. By embracing practices that minimize waste, families can instill values of responsibility and resourcefulness in their children, ensuring that the next generation is equipped to make informed decisions about food and waste. Through conscious choices in the kitchen, families can contribute to a greener planet while enjoying the myriad benefits of nutritious, flavorful meals.

Understanding Sustainable Ingredients

Understanding sustainable ingredients is essential for families looking to create a greener kitchen while also prioritizing health. Sustainable ingredients are those that are produced in ways that do not deplete natural resources, protect ecosystems, and promote overall well-being for both consumers and producers. This concept encourages the use of foods that are organic, ethically sourced, and minimally processed. By choosing sustainable ingredients, families can contribute to environmental conservation, support local economies, and improve their own health through nutrient-rich options.

One of the cornerstones of sustainable cooking is opting for locally sourced superfoods. These ingredients are often fresher, tastier, and more nutritious compared to those that have traveled long distances. By supporting local farmers and markets, families not only reduce their carbon footprint but also foster community relationships. Seasonal produce, such as fruits and vegetables, can be incorporated into meals to enhance flavor and nutrient density while minimizing waste. This approach encourages families to plan their meals around what is available locally, promoting a connection with the earth and the cycles of nature.

Plant-based meal prep is another vital aspect of utilizing sustainable ingredients. Transitioning to a plant-based diet, even partially, can significantly lower environmental impact by reducing reliance on animal agriculture, which is resource-intensive. Families can explore various plant-based proteins, such as legumes, grains, and nuts, which are not only sustainable but also packed with essential nutrients. Preparing meals in advance allows families to make informed choices about their nutrition and waste reduction, ensuring that wholesome, plant-based options are always on hand.

Eco-friendly packaging solutions play an important role in the sustainability of food choices. When selecting ingredients, families should consider products that come in minimal or recyclable packaging. This reduces the amount of waste generated in the kitchen and contributes to a circular economy. Many local markets now offer bulk bins where families can purchase items without packaging, further decreasing their environmental footprint. Educating children about the importance of sustainable packaging can foster a sense of responsibility and encourage them to be mindful consumers.

Incorporating herbal and medicinal foods into daily cooking can enhance the health benefits of meals while remaining sustainable. Herbs and spices not only add flavor but also offer numerous health benefits, such as anti-inflammatory properties and antioxidants. Families can grow their own herbs at home, which requires little space and provides fresh ingredients for cooking. Additionally, creating nutrient-dense smoothies using locally sourced fruits, vegetables, and herbal supplements can serve as a delicious and convenient way to boost health while adhering to sustainable practices. By understanding and embracing sustainable ingredients, families can lead healthier lives and contribute to a more sustainable world.

Benefits of a Greener Kitchen

A greener kitchen offers numerous benefits that extend beyond simply reducing waste. For families, adopting sustainable practices can lead to healthier eating habits and improved overall well-being. By focusing on plant-based meal preparation, families can incorporate a wider variety of fruits, vegetables, and whole grains into their diets. This not only enhances nutritional intake but also fosters a positive relationship with food. Engaging children and teens in the kitchen can empower them to make informed choices about what they eat, setting the stage for lifelong healthy habits.

Sourcing locally grown superfoods is another significant advantage of a greener kitchen. By purchasing ingredients from local farmers and markets, families can ensure that their food is fresh, seasonal, and free from harmful preservatives. This practice not only supports the local economy but also reduces the carbon footprint associated with long-distance food transport. Additionally, local produce often contains more nutrients due to its freshness, providing families with a greater range of vitamins and minerals essential for health.

Eco-friendly packaging solutions play a crucial role in creating a greener kitchen. By opting for bulk purchasing and reusable containers, families can significantly reduce the amount of plastic waste generated in their homes. Encouraging the use of glass jars, beeswax wraps, and compostable materials not only minimizes environmental impact but also promotes a culture of sustainability within the household. These small changes can lead to substantial reductions in waste over time, inspiring family members to adopt eco-conscious behaviors in other areas of their lives.

Nutrient-dense smoothie recipes are a fantastic way to incorporate more plant-based foods into daily meals while minimizing waste. By utilizing overripe fruits and leftover vegetables, families can create delicious and nutritious smoothies that would otherwise go to waste. This method not only helps reduce food waste but also encourages creativity in the kitchen. By experimenting with different combinations of ingredients, family members can explore new flavors and textures, making healthy eating enjoyable and accessible for everyone.

Lastly, low-waste cooking techniques, such as composting food scraps and using every part of an ingredient, reinforce the benefits of a greener kitchen. Families can learn to repurpose vegetable peels, stems, and other leftovers into stocks or broths, maximizing the use of their ingredients. This not only reduces waste but also promotes mindfulness around food consumption. By instilling these practices in young cooks, families can cultivate a sustainable mindset that prioritizes resourcefulness and respect for the environment, ultimately leading to a healthier lifestyle for all.

Chapter 2: Plant-Based Meal Prep

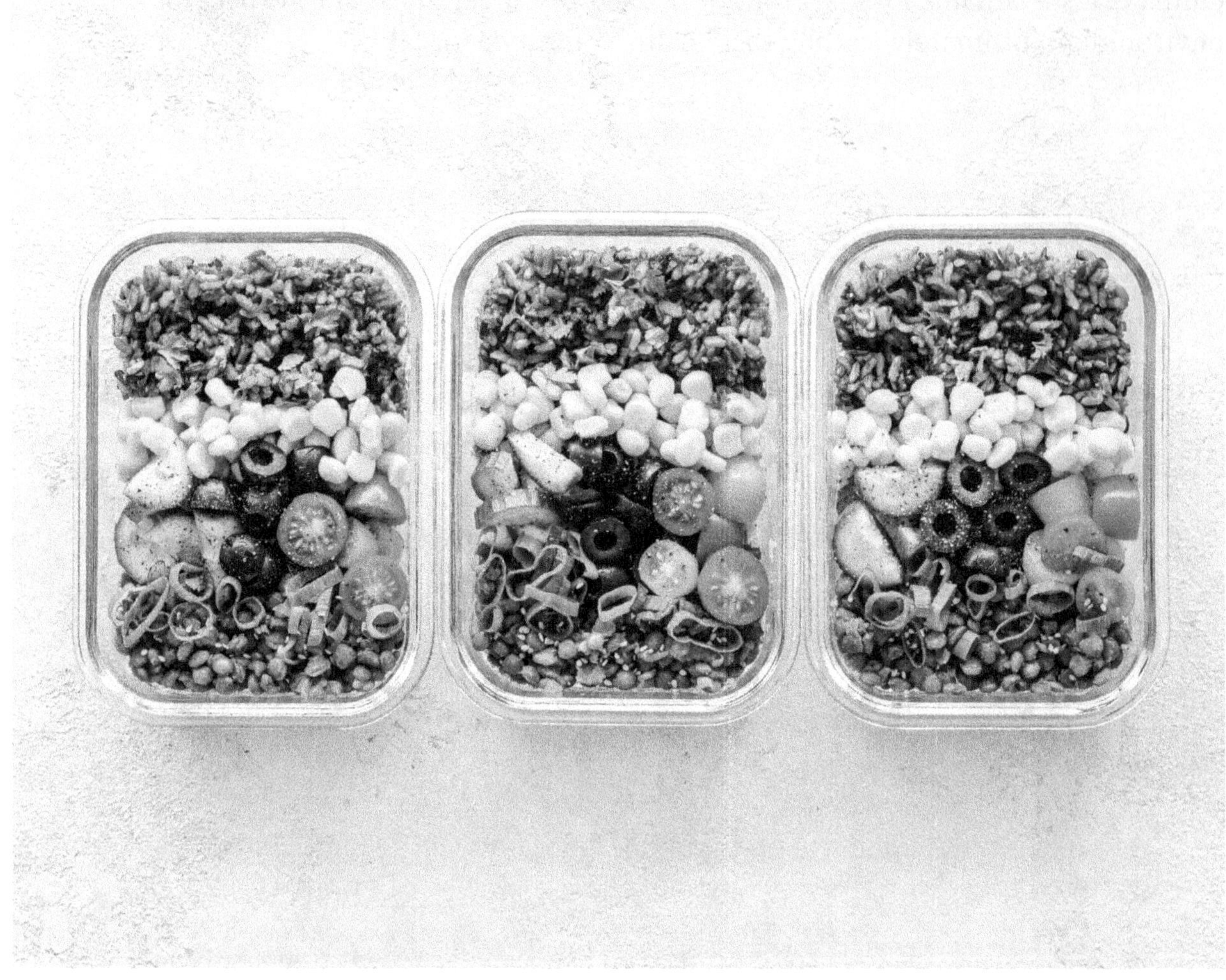

Basics of Plant-Based Cooking

Plant-based cooking revolves around the use of fruits, vegetables, grains, legumes, nuts, and seeds, forming the foundation of a sustainable and health-conscious diet. Families looking to embrace this culinary approach will find that it not only promotes wellness but also aligns with environmentally friendly practices. Incorporating a variety of plant-based foods can enhance nutritional intake while reducing reliance on animal products, which often have a larger carbon footprint. Understanding the basics of plant-based cooking paves the way for creating delicious and nutritious meals that appeal to all family members.

One key aspect of plant-based cooking is the emphasis on whole foods. Whole foods are minimally processed and retain their natural nutrients, making them ideal for boosting health. Families can focus on incorporating seasonal produce, which is often fresher and more flavorful, while supporting local farmers. This approach not only reduces waste associated with packaging but also fosters a connection to the community food system. By planning meals around what is in season, families can enjoy a diverse array of nutrients and flavors throughout the year.

Meal preparation plays a crucial role in plant-based cooking, especially for busy families and teen cooks. Planning and preparing meals in advance can help streamline the cooking process and minimize food waste. By batch cooking grains, legumes, and roasted vegetables, families can create a variety of dishes with minimal effort during the week. Utilizing eco-friendly packaging solutions, such as reusable containers, encourages sustainable practices and reduces single-use plastics. This approach not only promotes healthier eating habits but also instills valuable cooking skills in young chefs.

Nutrient-dense smoothies are another fantastic way to incorporate plant-based ingredients into daily meals. These blended beverages can serve as quick breakfasts, snacks, or even light lunches, packed with vitamins, minerals, and antioxidants. Families can experiment with different combinations of fruits, vegetables, nuts, and seeds to create smoothies that cater to their individual tastes and nutritional needs. Adding superfoods like spinach, chia seeds, or nut butters can enhance the nutrient profile, making smoothies a versatile and easy option for health-conscious households.

Finally, low-waste cooking techniques are integral to the philosophy of plant-based cooking. Families can minimize waste by utilizing vegetable scraps to make broths or composting organic materials. Learning to repurpose leftovers into new meals, such as transforming roasted vegetables into hearty soups or using overripe fruits in baking, can significantly reduce food waste. By adopting these practices, families not only contribute to a more sustainable kitchen but also foster creativity in their cooking, turning what might be seen as waste into delicious and nutritious meals.

Meal Planning for Busy Families

Meal planning is an essential strategy for busy families aiming to maintain a sustainable and health-conscious kitchen. With the hustle and bustle of daily life, it can be challenging to prioritize nutritious meals while minimizing waste. By dedicating time each week to plan meals, families can streamline grocery shopping, reduce food waste, and ensure that nutritious, plant-based options are readily available. This proactive approach not only supports healthier eating habits but also fosters a culture of sustainability within the household.

To begin effective meal planning, families should assess their schedules for the week ahead. Identifying busy days allows for the preparation of quick, nutrient-dense meals that can be made in advance. For instance, batch-cooking grains and legumes can serve as a foundation for various dishes throughout the week. Incorporating locally sourced superfoods into these meals enhances both the nutritional value and the environmental impact of the family's diet, promoting a reduced carbon footprint through the support of local farmers.

When selecting recipes, families can focus on seasonal produce that is not only fresher but also more affordable. Planning meals around these ingredients encourages creativity in the kitchen and reduces reliance on out-of-season, imported foods that often come in eco-unfriendly packaging. Utilizing low-waste cooking techniques, such as making stocks from vegetable scraps or repurposing leftovers, further complements the goal of minimizing waste. Families can also engage their children in this process, teaching them about the importance of sustainability and how to make conscious food choices.

A vital component of meal planning is the preparation of nutrient-dense snacks and smoothies. By incorporating a variety of fruits, vegetables, and herbs into these recipes, families can craft quick, healthful options that are perfect for on-the-go lifestyles. Smoothies can be made in bulk and stored in reusable containers, ensuring easy access to wholesome nutrition. Additionally, experimenting with herbal and medicinal foods can enhance both flavor and health benefits, offering natural boosts to the immune system and overall wellness.

Lastly, eco-friendly packaging solutions play a crucial role in maintaining the sustainability of meal planning. Families can invest in reusable containers and storage options that reduce single-use plastics. When shopping, opting for bulk items or choosing zero-waste stores can significantly cut down on packaging waste. By integrating these practices into their meal planning routine, families not only nourish their bodies with wholesome, plant-based foods but also contribute to a greener planet, reinforcing the idea that every small effort counts in the pursuit of a sustainable future.

Batch Cooking Techniques

Batch cooking is a practical approach that allows families to prepare meals in large quantities, reducing both time spent in the kitchen and food waste. By dedicating a specific day each week to cook in bulk, families can create a variety of dishes that can be stored for later use. This method not only promotes efficiency but also encourages the use of sustainable and health-conscious ingredients, such as plant-based proteins and locally sourced produce. When planned thoughtfully, batch cooking can help families maintain a nutritious diet while minimizing their environmental impact.

To begin batch cooking effectively, it is essential to establish a menu that incorporates nutrient-dense ingredients. Focus on seasonal vegetables, whole grains, and legumes that are not only healthy but also support local farmers. By choosing ingredients that are in season, families can enjoy fresher flavors and reduce the carbon footprint associated with transporting food long distances. Additionally, incorporating superfoods such as quinoa, lentils, and leafy greens can enhance the nutritional profile of meals, ensuring that families consume a well-rounded diet.

Next, organizing cooking sessions can streamline the process. Gather ingredients in advance and allocate specific times for each stage of cooking. This could involve roasting vegetables, simmering soups, or preparing grains simultaneously. Utilizing multi-purpose kitchen tools, like slow cookers or pressure cookers, can significantly reduce cooking times and energy usage. As families create different dishes, they can portion out meals into eco-friendly containers or jars, making it easy to grab a nutritious option during busy days or when mealtime approaches.

Storage techniques also play a crucial role in batch cooking. To maximize freshness and reduce waste, families should focus on using glass containers or reusable silicone bags for storing prepared meals. Clearly labeling each container with the date and contents can help in tracking freshness and ensuring meals are consumed in a timely manner. For items that may spoil faster, such as salads or delicate greens, consider preparing components separately and combining them just before serving. This method retains flavor and texture while minimizing waste.

Finally, batch cooking opens the door to creative meal combinations and experimentation with flavors. Families can use leftover ingredients from one dish to enhance another, allowing for innovative recipes that keep mealtimes exciting. For instance, roasted vegetables from one meal can be transformed into a flavorful smoothie or blended into a sauce for pasta. This creativity not only reduces food waste but also encourages families to explore new culinary techniques and incorporate medicinal herbs into their cooking. Ultimately, batch cooking fosters a sustainable kitchen environment, empowering families to embrace healthy habits while caring for the planet.

Chapter 3: Locally Sourced Superfoods

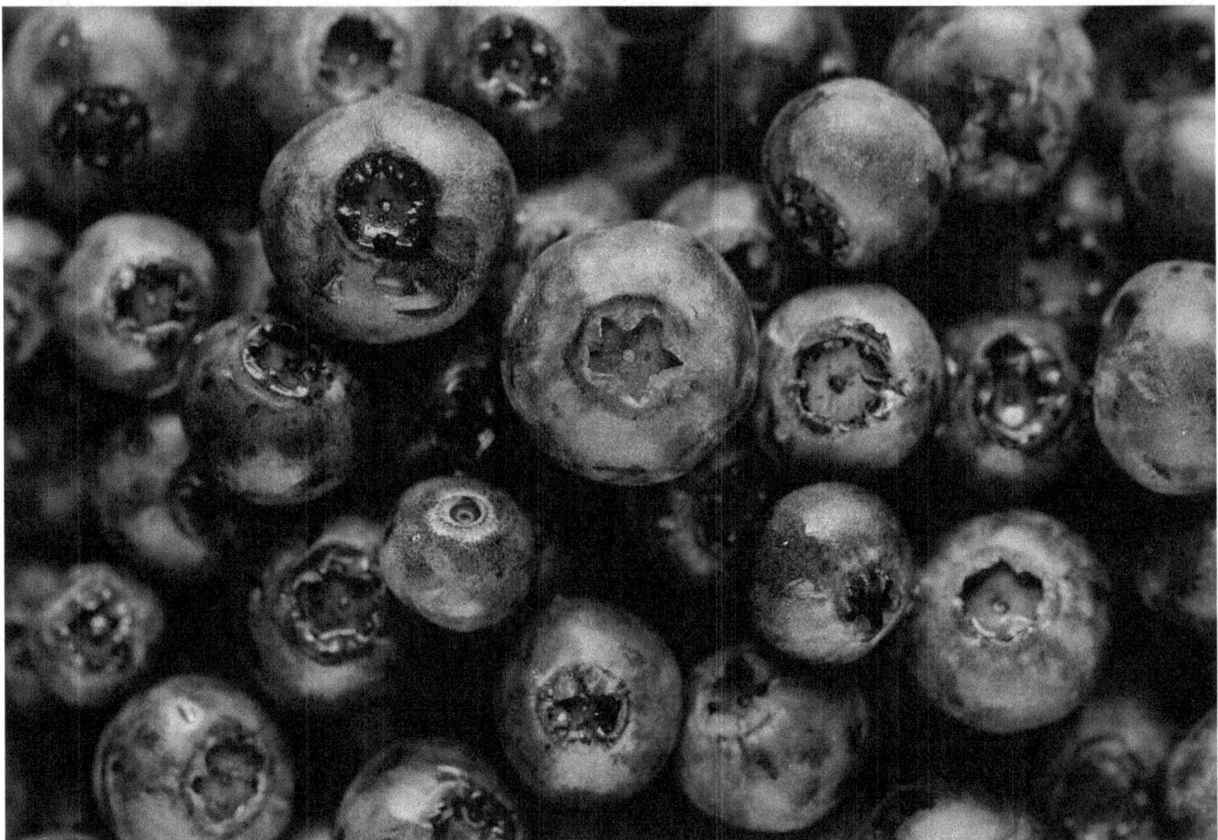

Identifying Local Superfoods

Identifying local superfoods involves understanding the nutritional powerhouses that grow in your region, often packed with nutrients and flavor. Superfoods are typically classified as nutrient-dense foods that can offer health benefits beyond basic nutrition. They include fruits, vegetables, grains, nuts, and herbs that are rich in vitamins, minerals, and antioxidants. By focusing on local varieties, families can not only elevate their meals but also support local farmers, reduce their carbon footprint, and promote sustainable eating habits.

The first step in identifying local superfoods is to research what is grown in your area. This can be done through local farmers' markets, community-supported agriculture (CSA) programs, and agricultural extension offices. Seasonal produce guides can also be valuable resources, helping you understand what fruits and vegetables are at their peak in your region. For instance, leafy greens like kale and spinach, berries like blueberries and strawberries, and legumes such as beans and lentils may be readily available and highly nutritious. Knowing what is local and seasonal can guide your meal planning and grocery shopping, allowing you to make informed choices.

Engaging with local agriculture not only benefits your health but also your community. Many local farms prioritize sustainable practices, which means the produce is often fresher and free from excessive chemicals. By choosing locally sourced superfoods, families can support these eco-friendly practices and encourage biodiversity in their region. Additionally, local foods often have higher nutrient retention compared to imported items, which can lose nutrients during transportation. This makes a compelling case for incorporating local superfoods into your diet, as they can deliver maximum health benefits.

Incorporating local superfoods into your meals can be both fun and creative. Experimenting with different cooking techniques can enhance the flavors and textures of these nutrient-dense ingredients. Consider making smoothies packed with local fruits and greens, using herbs from your backyard to add freshness, or preparing a colorful grain bowl featuring seasonal vegetables. These meals can be not only satisfying but also visually appealing, making them a hit with family members of all ages. The goal is to inspire young cooks and families to explore their local food landscape and create delicious, healthful dishes.

Finally, documenting your discoveries and recipes can contribute to a greater movement toward sustainable cooking practices. Sharing your experiences with local superfoods through social media or community forums can inspire others to join in on the journey toward healthier eating habits. By identifying and utilizing local superfoods, families become part of a larger effort to promote sustainability in food systems. This not only benefits individual health but also supports the planet, ensuring future generations can enjoy the bounty of local produce.

Seasonal Eating and Its Benefits

Seasonal eating refers to the practice of consuming fruits and vegetables that are harvested during their natural growing seasons. This approach not only aligns with nature's cycles but also promotes a sustainable lifestyle. By choosing seasonal produce, families can enjoy fresher ingredients that are often more nutrient-dense. Seasonal foods are typically harvested at their peak ripeness, ensuring that they are packed with flavor and essential vitamins and minerals. This practice encourages families to connect with the local food system and supports local farmers, reducing the carbon footprint associated with long-distance transportation of food.

One of the primary benefits of seasonal eating is the positive impact it has on health. Seasonal produce tends to be more vibrant and flavorful, which can make meals more enjoyable and satisfying. For health-conscious cooks, incorporating a variety of seasonal fruits and vegetables into meal prep can lead to a more diverse intake of nutrients. Eating a wide range of produce helps to ensure that families receive the necessary vitamins, minerals, and antioxidants. Moreover, seasonal eating encourages the consumption of whole, unprocessed foods, reducing the reliance on packaged items that may contain preservatives and artificial ingredients.

In addition to health benefits, seasonal eating can also lead to significant cost savings. When fruits and vegetables are in season, they are generally more abundant and therefore more affordable. Families can take advantage of local farmers' markets or community-supported agriculture (CSA) programs to access fresh produce at lower prices. This not only supports local economies but also promotes the consumption of organic and sustainably grown foods. By planning meals around what is in season, families can save money while enjoying high-quality ingredients that are better for their health and the environment.

Seasonal eating also fosters creativity in the kitchen. Families and teen cooks can experiment with a variety of ingredients that change throughout the year. This encourages the exploration of new recipes and cooking techniques, making meal preparation a fun and engaging family activity. Using seasonal ingredients can inspire families to create dishes that highlight the unique flavors of each season, from hearty winter stews to refreshing summer salads. This approach not only reduces waste by utilizing ingredients at their peak but also enhances the cooking experience by incorporating fresh, local flavors.

Lastly, adopting seasonal eating habits can contribute to a greater awareness of food sustainability. As families learn about the benefits of eating seasonally, they become more conscious of their food choices and their impact on the environment. This awareness can lead to more eco-friendly practices in the kitchen, such as composting scraps, utilizing eco-friendly packaging solutions, and minimizing food waste. By prioritizing seasonal ingredients, families can cultivate a deeper connection to their food, promote a healthier lifestyle, and contribute to a more sustainable food system for future generations.

Incorporating Superfoods into Family Meals

Incorporating superfoods into family meals can be a transformative experience for both health and sustainability. Superfoods, often rich in nutrients and antioxidants, can enhance the nutritional value of everyday dishes while also supporting local agriculture. Families looking to adopt a healthier lifestyle can start by integrating these ingredients into meals that everyone will enjoy. The key is to find superfoods that are versatile and appealing to all ages, ensuring that the entire family benefits from their health properties without feeling overwhelmed by drastic changes in their diets.

One effective approach is to include superfoods in familiar recipes. For instance, adding spinach or kale to smoothies, soups, or sauces can significantly boost their nutrient content without altering the taste. These leafy greens are packed with vitamins A, C, and K, making them excellent choices for enhancing family meals. Utilizing local superfoods such as berries, nuts, or seeds can also provide essential nutrients. Purchasing these ingredients from local farmers' markets not only supports the community but also reduces the carbon footprint associated with transporting food over long distances.

Incorporating superfoods into meals can also inspire creative cooking techniques that minimize waste. Families can use vegetable scraps to make nutrient-rich broths or smoothies, ensuring that every part of the food is utilized. For example, carrot tops can be blended into pesto or added to salads for an extra kick of flavor and nutrients. This approach not only elevates the meals but also instills a sense of resourcefulness in young cooks, teaching them the importance of reducing waste in the kitchen.

Another way to engage family members in incorporating superfoods is through meal prep activities. Involving children and teens in planning and preparing meals can foster an appreciation for healthy eating and sustainable practices. Designating a day for family meal prep, where everyone can contribute by chopping vegetables, blending smoothies, or creating snack packs with superfoods, can be both educational and fun. This hands-on experience allows young cooks to learn about superfoods, their benefits, and how to incorporate them into various dishes.

Finally, it is essential to emphasize the importance of eco-friendly packaging solutions when buying superfoods. Choosing bulk bins, reusable containers, and local products can significantly decrease waste associated with food packaging. By consciously selecting ingredients that come with minimal or no packaging, families can enjoy superfoods while promoting sustainability. This mindful approach not only nourishes the body but also cultivates a deeper connection to the environment, encouraging a greener lifestyle for everyone in the family.

Chapter 4: Eco-Friendly Packaging Solutions

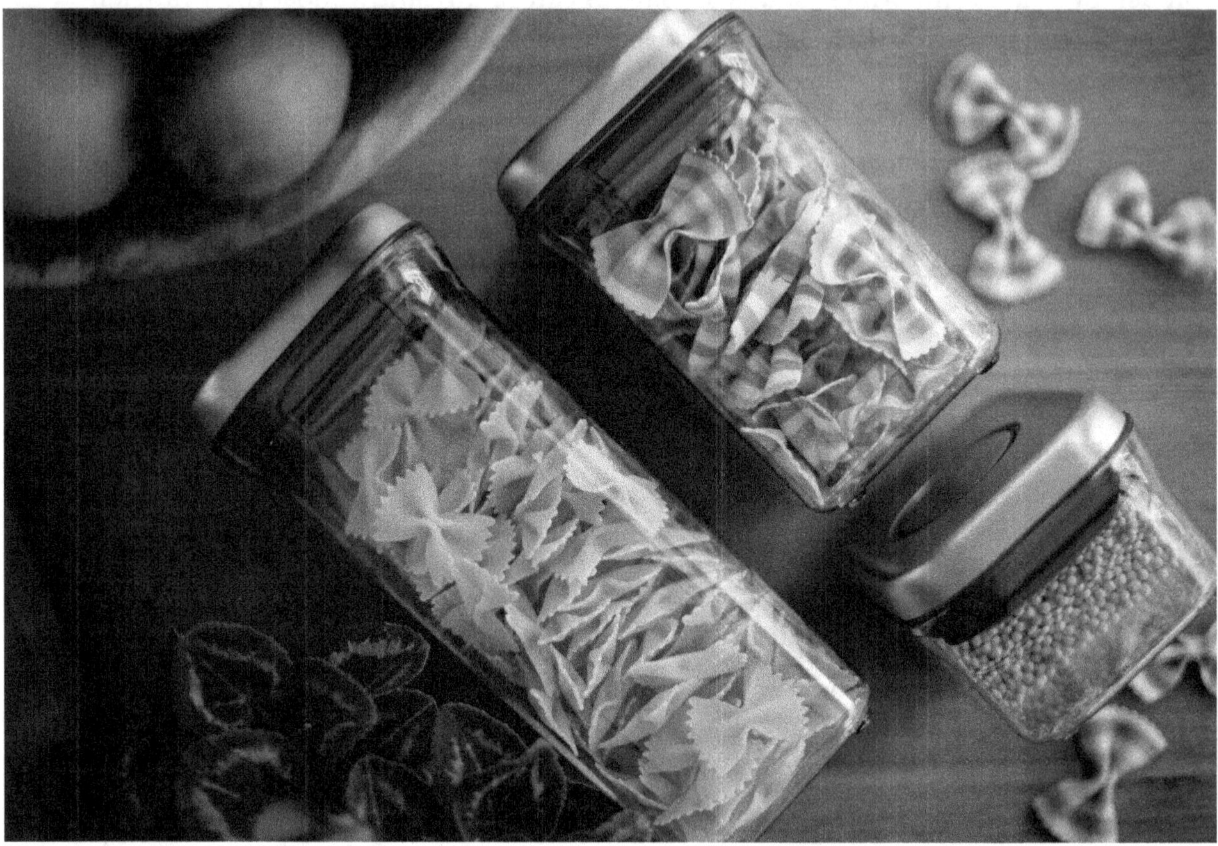

Understanding Packaging Waste

Understanding packaging waste is crucial for families striving to minimize their environmental footprint while maintaining a healthy kitchen. In our modern food system, packaging plays a significant role in convenience and preservation, but it also contributes substantially to the waste generated in households. Understanding the types of packaging materials and their environmental impact can help families make more informed choices, encouraging a shift toward sustainable alternatives that align with eco-friendly cooking practices.

Many common packaging materials, such as plastic, cardboard, and styrofoam, have different lifespans and disposal challenges. Plastics, while lightweight and versatile, can take hundreds of years to decompose and often end up in landfills or the ocean, where they contribute to pollution and harm marine life. Cardboard and paper, on the other hand, are more biodegradable but can still pose issues if they are coated with plastic or treated with chemicals. Families should be aware of these distinctions to better navigate their grocery shopping and meal prep, opting for products with minimal or recyclable packaging whenever possible.

Transitioning to sustainable packaging solutions can significantly reduce a family's overall waste. One practical approach is to choose products packaged in glass, metal, or compostable materials. These alternatives are usually more environmentally friendly and often offer better protection for food. Additionally, many local markets and grocery stores now provide options for bulk buying, allowing families to use their own reusable containers, further decreasing the amount of packaging waste produced. This practice not only supports sustainable purchasing habits but also encourages mindful consumption of food resources.

Incorporating low-waste cooking techniques can further complement efforts to minimize packaging waste. Families can explore creative ways to utilize food scraps, such as turning vegetable peelings into broths or using overripe fruits in smoothies. This not only maximizes the use of the ingredients purchased but also reduces the need for additional packaging that comes with buying pre-packaged food items. Cooking with a focus on reducing waste encourages a more holistic approach to meal preparation, fostering creativity and resourcefulness in the kitchen.

Ultimately, understanding packaging waste and its implications is an essential step in building a greener family kitchen. By being informed about the materials we encounter and making conscious choices about food packaging, families can play an active role in reducing their environmental impact. This newfound awareness, combined with sustainable cooking practices, empowers families to create delicious, health-conscious meals while contributing to a healthier planet for future generations.

Sustainable Alternatives to Common Packaging

The growing awareness of environmental issues has led many families to seek sustainable alternatives to common packaging materials, which often contribute to pollution and waste. Traditional packaging, such as plastic, poses significant threats to our ecosystems and health. By choosing eco-friendly options, families can not only reduce their carbon footprint but also embrace a healthier lifestyle. Sustainable alternatives are becoming increasingly accessible, making it easier for families to adopt practices that promote environmental stewardship while preparing nutritious meals.

One popular alternative to plastic packaging is beeswax wraps. Made from cotton fabric infused with beeswax, these wraps are biodegradable and can be reused multiple times. They provide an excellent way to cover food items, wrap sandwiches, or store leftovers without the harmful effects of plastic. Families can also create their own wraps using natural ingredients, allowing for customization in size and design. This not only reduces waste but also engages children in the kitchen, teaching them about sustainability and creativity.

Glass containers offer another practical solution for food storage. Unlike plastic, glass is non-toxic and does not leach chemicals into food, making it a healthier choice for meal prep. They are durable, reusable, and recyclable, ensuring that they contribute to a low-waste lifestyle. Families can invest in a variety of sizes for different uses, from storing bulk grains to packing lunches. Opting for glass containers encourages mindful eating and reduces the temptation to rely on single-use plastics for convenience.

For those who enjoy smoothies and nutrient-dense recipes, consider using compostable cups or jars for serving. Many brands now offer biodegradable options made from plant-based materials, which break down naturally and do not contribute to landfill waste. This is particularly important for families who frequently prepare smoothies or other beverages, as it allows them to enjoy their creations without guilt. Additionally, utilizing reusable straws made from bamboo or stainless steel can further minimize waste while adding an element of style to their meals.

Lastly, exploring local farmers' markets can provide families with fresh produce that often comes with minimal packaging. Many vendors offer bulk items or encourage customers to bring their own containers for purchases, fostering a community-oriented approach to sustainable eating. By sourcing ingredients locally, families not only support their local economy but also reduce the environmental impact associated with transporting goods over long distances. This connection to local food sources reinforces the values of sustainability and health, creating a positive cycle that benefits both the family and the planet.

Tips for Reducing Kitchen Waste

Reducing kitchen waste is a crucial step toward creating a more sustainable family kitchen. Families and cooks who prioritize health and eco-friendliness can adopt simple practices to minimize waste while still enjoying nutritious meals. One effective method is to plan meals ahead of time. By creating a weekly menu based on what you already have in your pantry and fridge, you can prevent overbuying and ensure that all ingredients are used before they spoil. This approach not only cuts down on waste but also helps save money and time.

Another key strategy is to repurpose food scraps. Many families throw away vegetable peels, stems, and herb trimmings without realizing their potential. For example, vegetable scraps can be simmered to create a flavorful broth, while herb stems can be blended into sauces or pesto. Additionally, fruit peels can be used in smoothies or as natural flavor enhancers in water. By getting creative with leftovers and scraps, you not only reduce waste but also enrich your meals with new flavors and nutrients.

Emphasizing plant-based meal prep can also significantly lower kitchen waste. Plant-based diets often involve ingredients that can be utilized in multiple ways. For instance, a single batch of quinoa can be transformed into a salad, grain bowl, or soup throughout the week. Focusing on versatile ingredients encourages the use of all parts of the produce while providing nourishing meals for the family. Additionally, incorporating locally sourced superfoods into your cooking not only supports regional farmers but also ensures fresher ingredients that have a longer shelf life.

Eco-friendly packaging solutions play a vital role in waste reduction as well. Families should consider investing in reusable containers for storing leftovers and buying in bulk to minimize packaging waste. When shopping, choose products with minimal or compostable packaging, and bring your own bags to the store. This conscious effort not only reduces plastic waste but also aligns with a commitment to sustainability. Moreover, teaching teens about the importance of eco-friendly practices fosters a sense of responsibility and encourages them to make mindful choices in the kitchen.

Finally, integrating low-waste cooking techniques can transform how your family approaches meal preparation. Techniques like batch cooking, where larger quantities are made and portioned for future meals, help prevent food from going stale or spoiling. Creating nutrient-dense smoothie recipes using overripe fruits and vegetables is another great way to reduce waste while providing your family with healthy options. By adopting these tips, families can cultivate a kitchen environment that prioritizes sustainability, health, and creativity, ultimately contributing to a greener planet.

Chapter 5: Nutrient-Dense Smoothie Recipes

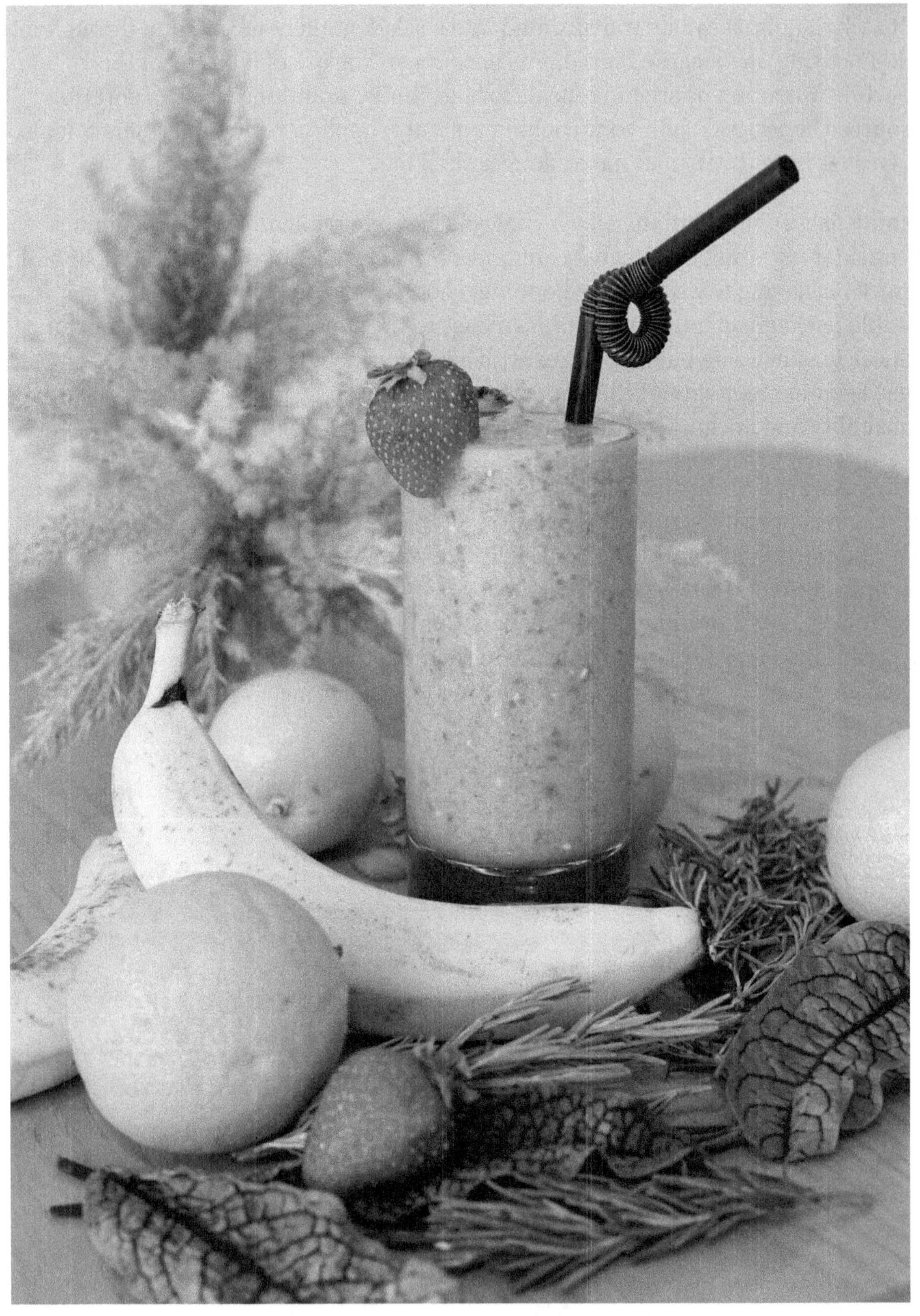

Building a Balanced Smoothie

Building a balanced smoothie is an essential skill for families seeking nutritious, sustainable meals that cater to various dietary preferences. A well-crafted smoothie can serve as a quick breakfast, a wholesome snack, or a post-workout refreshment. The key to creating a balanced smoothie lies in the thoughtful selection of ingredients that not only provide essential nutrients but also minimize waste. By focusing on locally sourced superfoods and seasonal produce, families can support their local economy while ensuring they consume the freshest ingredients available.

To create a nutrient-dense smoothie, start with a solid base. Leafy greens like spinach, kale, or Swiss chard are excellent choices. These greens are packed with vitamins, minerals, and antioxidants, making them a powerhouse of nutrition. Choosing organic or locally sourced greens can enhance the sustainability of your smoothie, reducing the carbon footprint associated with transportation. Additionally, incorporating these greens can help families utilize surplus produce that might otherwise go to waste, thereby promoting a low-waste cooking technique.

Next, add a source of healthy fats to enhance the smoothie's texture and nutritional profile. Ingredients such as avocados, nut butters, or seeds like chia or flax provide essential fatty acids that support brain health and keep you feeling full longer. These ingredients can also help balance the natural sugars found in fruits, preventing blood sugar spikes. By selecting organic or bulk options, families can reduce packaging waste and contribute to eco-friendly practices in their kitchen.

Fruits are the star of any smoothie, providing natural sweetness and vibrant flavor. Opt for a variety of fruits, including berries, bananas, or seasonal fruits that are locally available. Berries, in particular, are rich in antioxidants and can often be sourced from local farms. To further reduce waste, consider using frozen fruits, which often have a longer shelf life and can be made from surplus produce that might otherwise spoil. This approach not only helps in minimizing waste but also ensures that your smoothie remains refreshing and nutrient-rich year-round.

Lastly, enhance your smoothie with herbal and medicinal foods to boost its health benefits. Ingredients like ginger, turmeric, or even fresh herbs such as mint or basil can provide unique flavors and added nutritional value. These herbs are often easy to grow at home, encouraging families to cultivate their own ingredients and reduce reliance on store-bought options. By employing eco-friendly packaging solutions, such as reusable containers for smoothie prep, families can further embrace a sustainable lifestyle while enjoying delicious, health-conscious smoothies.

Creative Ingredient Combinations

Creative ingredient combinations can transform your cooking, allowing for exciting flavors while embracing sustainability and health. By thinking outside the box and exploring unusual pairings, families can minimize food waste and create nutrient-dense meals that are both delicious and nourishing. This approach encourages using ingredients that might typically be overlooked, such as vegetable scraps, herbs, and grains, fostering a habit of resourcefulness in the kitchen.

One effective way to explore creative combinations is through the use of local superfoods. Integrating seasonal produce not only supports local farmers but also enhances the nutritional profile of meals. For instance, pairing kale, a nutrient powerhouse, with sweet potatoes brings together a delightful contrast in textures and flavors, while also providing a rich source of vitamins and minerals. Experimenting with local ingredients encourages families to discover new tastes, making healthy eating an enjoyable adventure.

Plant-based meal prep is another avenue where creativity can shine. Combining legumes, grains, and vegetables can lead to satisfying dishes filled with protein and fiber. A quinoa and black bean salad, for example, can be elevated with the addition of roasted seasonal vegetables and a citrus vinaigrette. These combinations not only reduce waste by utilizing leftovers but also create vibrant meals that appeal to both adults and teens, encouraging everyone to participate in the cooking process.

Herbs and spices play a crucial role in enhancing flavors, and they can be creatively paired with unusual ingredients to create memorable dishes. For instance, incorporating fresh mint into a smoothie with spinach and avocado not only adds a refreshing twist but also boosts the drink's nutrient content. By focusing on herbal and medicinal foods, families can also introduce their children to the health benefits of various plants, fostering a deeper understanding of food's impact on well-being.

Lastly, eco-friendly packaging solutions can complement these creative ingredient combinations by encouraging families to shop mindfully. Bulk buying and using reusable containers can reduce plastic waste while providing the opportunity to experiment with a variety of ingredients. By embracing low-waste cooking techniques, families can create innovative meals that reflect their values and inspire a more sustainable lifestyle. Through these practices, cooking becomes not only a means of sustenance but also a creative outlet that fosters family bonding and environmental awareness.

Smoothies for Different Dietary Needs

Smoothies are a versatile and nutritious option for families looking to meet various dietary needs while minimizing waste. By choosing the right ingredients, smoothies can cater to specific nutritional requirements such as gluten-free, dairy-free, or even low-sugar diets. Families can easily adapt recipes to incorporate local, seasonal produce, reducing environmental impact while supporting community farmers. This approach not only provides a healthful addition to meals but also promotes sustainable eating practices that can be enjoyed by the entire family.

For those following a plant-based diet, smoothies are a fantastic way to incorporate a variety of fruits, vegetables, and plant-based proteins. Ingredients like spinach, kale, and avocados offer a wealth of nutrients, while nut butters, seeds, and plant-based protein powders can enhance the smoothie's protein content. Families can take advantage of local superfoods such as hemp seeds and chia seeds, which are rich in omega-3 fatty acids and fiber, contributing to a balanced diet. This not only aligns with health goals but also supports sustainable farming practices.

Health-conscious cooks often seek to minimize added sugars in their diets, and smoothies provide an excellent opportunity to create naturally sweet blends without compromising on flavor. Using ripe fruits such as bananas, mangoes, or berries can impart sweetness while providing essential vitamins and antioxidants. Additionally, incorporating ingredients like oats or unsweetened yogurt can create a satisfying texture. By experimenting with different flavor combinations, families can enjoy nutrient-dense smoothies that are both delicious and mindful of their sugar intake.

For those managing food allergies or intolerances, smoothies can be tailored to avoid problematic ingredients. For example, nut-free smoothies can be made using seeds or coconut milk as a creamy base. Utilizing alternative sweeteners such as dates or maple syrup can satisfy cravings without triggering allergies. Educating young cooks on the importance of reading labels and understanding food sourcing can empower them to make informed choices, ensuring that everyone in the family can enjoy smoothies that meet their individual health needs.

Lastly, eco-friendly packaging solutions play a crucial role in the preparation and consumption of smoothies. Families can invest in reusable containers for storing prepped smoothie ingredients, minimizing plastic waste. By creating a weekly smoothie prep routine, families can efficiently use up produce before it spoils, contributing to a lower overall waste footprint. This practice not only promotes sustainability but also encourages mindful eating habits, making smoothies an integral part of a greener family kitchen.

Chapter 6: Low-Waste Cooking Techniques

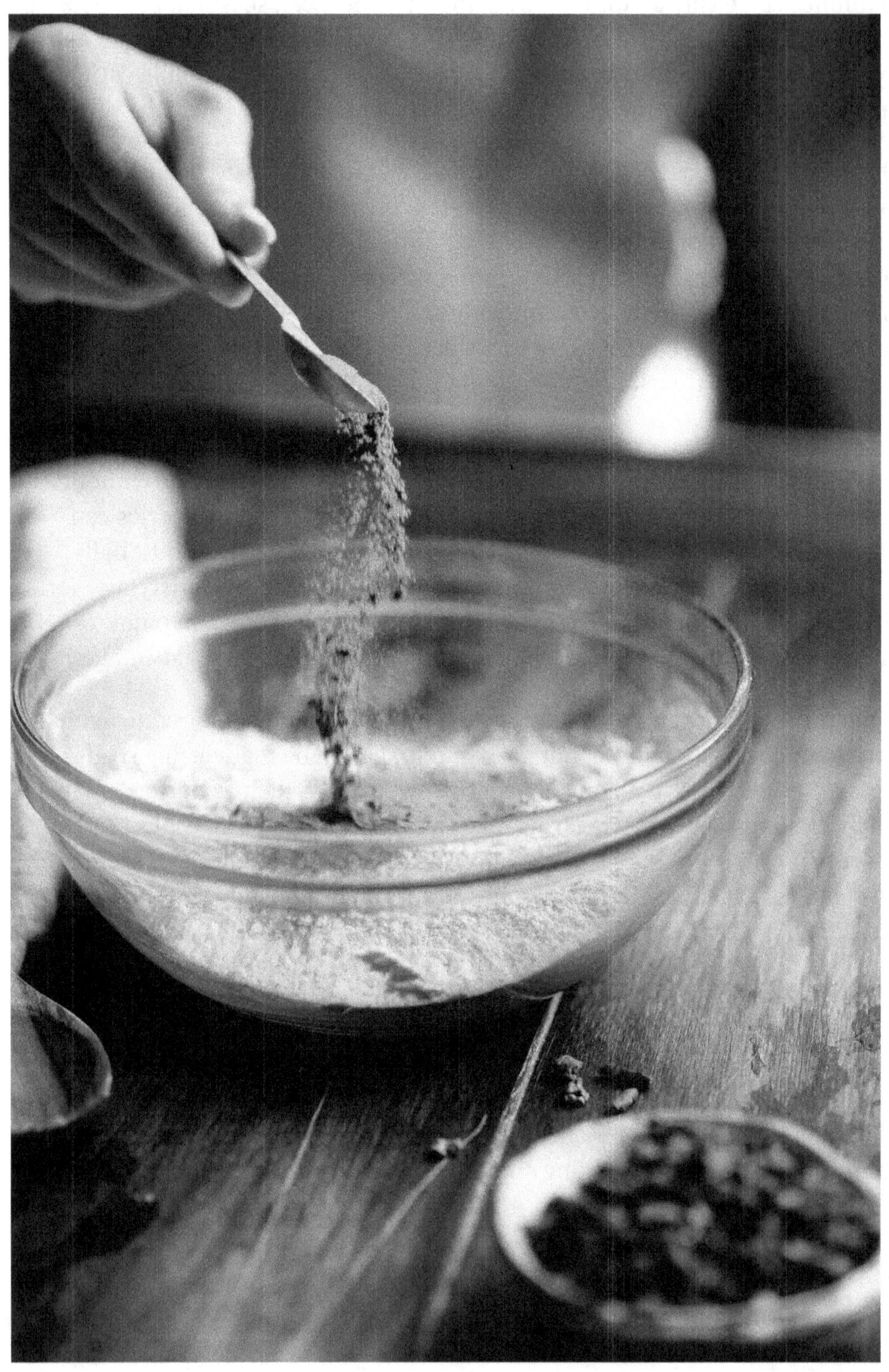

Utilizing Leftovers Effectively

Utilizing leftovers effectively is a cornerstone of sustainable cooking, allowing families to minimize waste while maximizing the nutritional benefits of their meals. With careful planning and creative thinking, leftover ingredients can be transformed into delicious new dishes, ensuring that nothing goes to waste. This not only helps the environment but also enables families to save money and time in the kitchen. By adopting a mindset that embraces leftovers, you can turn the remnants of one meal into the foundation for another, contributing to a greener family kitchen.

One effective strategy for utilizing leftovers is to incorporate them into new meals. For instance, roasted vegetables from a previous dinner can be blended into a nutritious soup or tossed into a grain bowl. Similarly, leftover grains like quinoa or brown rice can serve as a base for salads or stir-fries, adding both texture and nutrients. This approach not only enhances the flavors of your new dishes but also reduces the likelihood of food spoilage. By being resourceful with what you have, you can create a diverse array of meals that keep your family engaged and excited about eating.

Additionally, leftovers can be a great opportunity to experiment with plant-based recipes. Consider using leftover beans or lentils to whip up a hearty veggie burger or mixing them into a smoothie for an unexpected protein boost. Using vegetable scraps from meal prep, such as carrot tops or celery leaves, can also introduce unique flavors into smoothies or pestos. This approach not only utilizes what is often discarded but also introduces your family to new tastes and textures, promoting a more adventurous and health-conscious dining experience.

Eco-friendly packaging solutions also play a crucial role in effectively utilizing leftovers. Investing in reusable containers can help store leftovers properly, maintaining their freshness and preventing spoilage. When packing lunches or storing meals for the week, opt for glass jars or silicone bags that are not only sustainable but also keep food secure. Labeling these containers with dates can ensure that you consume them within a safe timeframe, further reducing waste. This simple habit encourages families to be more mindful of their food consumption and storage practices.

Lastly, integrating herbal and medicinal foods into your leftover meals can elevate both their flavor and health benefits. Herbs such as parsley, cilantro, or basil can be used to freshen up a dish, while also adding valuable nutrients. For example, adding fresh herbs to a leftover grain salad can create a vibrant, nutrient-dense meal. Similarly, incorporating spices known for their medicinal properties can enhance the healthfulness of your leftovers. By focusing on these elements, you can turn ordinary meals into extraordinary culinary experiences that not only satisfy hunger but also contribute to your family's overall well-being.

Creative Uses for Kitchen Scraps

Kitchen scraps often end up in the trash, but with a little creativity, they can be transformed into valuable ingredients that enhance your meals, reduce waste, and contribute to a sustainable kitchen. Families can engage in fun cooking projects that not only teach children about the importance of minimizing waste but also encourage them to appreciate the full potential of their food. From vegetable peels to stale bread, many scraps can be repurposed into nutritious and delicious dishes, making them a fantastic resource for health-conscious cooks looking for plant-based meal prep ideas.

One common kitchen scrap that is often overlooked is vegetable peels. Instead of discarding potato, carrot, or beet peels, consider turning them into crispy snacks. Simply toss the peels with a bit of oil, salt, and your favorite spices, then bake them until crispy. This not only reduces waste but also provides a nutrient-dense alternative to store-bought snacks. Additionally, vegetable scraps can be used to create a rich vegetable broth. Save your onion skins, celery tops, and herb stems in a bag in the freezer, and when you're ready, simmer them in water to extract their flavors. This broth can be the base for soups, stews, and sauces, adding depth and nutrition to your family meals.

Herbs are another kitchen staple that can be utilized beyond their initial purpose. Stems from herbs like basil, cilantro, and parsley often go unused, yet they carry a robust flavor. These stems can be finely chopped and added to sauces, salads, or even blended into pesto for a vibrant twist. Additionally, if you find yourself with wilted herbs, consider making an infused oil or vinegar. Simply combine the herbs with oil or vinegar and let them steep for a few days. This not only enhances the flavor of your culinary creations but also offers a creative way to use ingredients that might otherwise be discarded.

Stale bread is a common occurrence in many households, but it can be easily repurposed into breadcrumbs, croutons, or even a savory bread pudding. By drying out stale bread and grinding it into breadcrumbs, you can create a versatile ingredient for coating vegetables or proteins, adding texture to dishes, or thickening soups. Croutons can be made by cubing the bread, tossing it with olive oil and seasoning, and then baking until golden. These crunchy additions can elevate salads and soups, ensuring that even the least desirable bread finds a purpose in your kitchen.

Finally, fruit scraps such as cores, peels, and overripe produce should not be overlooked. Apple cores and peels can be simmered with water to create a flavorful apple cider vinegar, while banana peels can be used to make a nutrient-rich smoothie or composted to enrich your garden soil. Overripe fruits can be transformed into jams, sauces, or even incorporated into baked goods, ensuring that nothing goes to waste. By embracing these creative uses for kitchen scraps, families can cultivate a low-waste cooking culture, fostering a deeper connection with their food and promoting a healthier, more sustainable lifestyle.

Cooking Methods That Minimize Waste

Cooking methods that minimize waste are essential for families looking to adopt sustainable practices in their kitchens. One effective technique is the use of whole ingredients, which encourages cooks to utilize every part of a fruit or vegetable. For instance, carrot tops can be blended into pesto, while broccoli stems can be peeled and sautéed. This approach not only reduces waste but also enhances the nutritional value of meals. By getting creative with leftovers and utilizing parts of ingredients that are often discarded, families can make the most of their grocery purchases and contribute to a more sustainable food system.

Another impactful method is batch cooking, which involves preparing larger quantities of food at once for later use. This technique minimizes food waste by ensuring that ingredients are fully utilized before they spoil. Families can plan meals around ingredients that have a shorter shelf life, such as fresh produce, and then store the cooked meals in eco-friendly packaging for later consumption. Additionally, batch cooking allows for the creation of nutrient-dense dishes that can be easily reheated, saving time and energy during busy weekdays. By embracing this method, families not only reduce waste but also streamline their meal preparation process.

Emphasizing plant-based meal prep is also a significant way to reduce waste in the kitchen. Plant-based diets tend to have a lower environmental impact and often involve ingredients that can be used in multiple dishes. For example, grains like quinoa or brown rice can serve as the base for several meals throughout the week. Utilizing seasonal and locally sourced superfoods further supports sustainability, as these ingredients typically require less transportation and are fresher, leading to less spoilage. By focusing on plant-based options, families can create diverse and healthy meals while minimizing their overall waste footprint.

Fermentation is another innovative cooking method that supports waste reduction. This technique transforms excess vegetables into nutrient-rich foods, such as kimchi or sauerkraut, extending their shelf life significantly. Families can engage their children in the fermentation process, turning it into a fun and educational activity. This not only promotes a zero-waste mindset but also introduces beneficial probiotics into the family diet. By learning to ferment, families can preserve surplus produce and create flavorful accompaniments to their meals, enhancing both taste and nutrition.

Lastly, incorporating zero-waste cooking techniques into everyday practices can make a substantial difference. Simple strategies such as composting food scraps, using reusable containers for storage, and planning meals around pantry staples can significantly reduce kitchen waste. Encouraging teens and younger family members to participate in these practices can foster a sense of responsibility and awareness about food sustainability. By adopting these mindful cooking methods, families can create a greener kitchen environment that not only benefits their health but also contributes positively to the planet.

Chapter 7: Herbal and Medicinal Foods

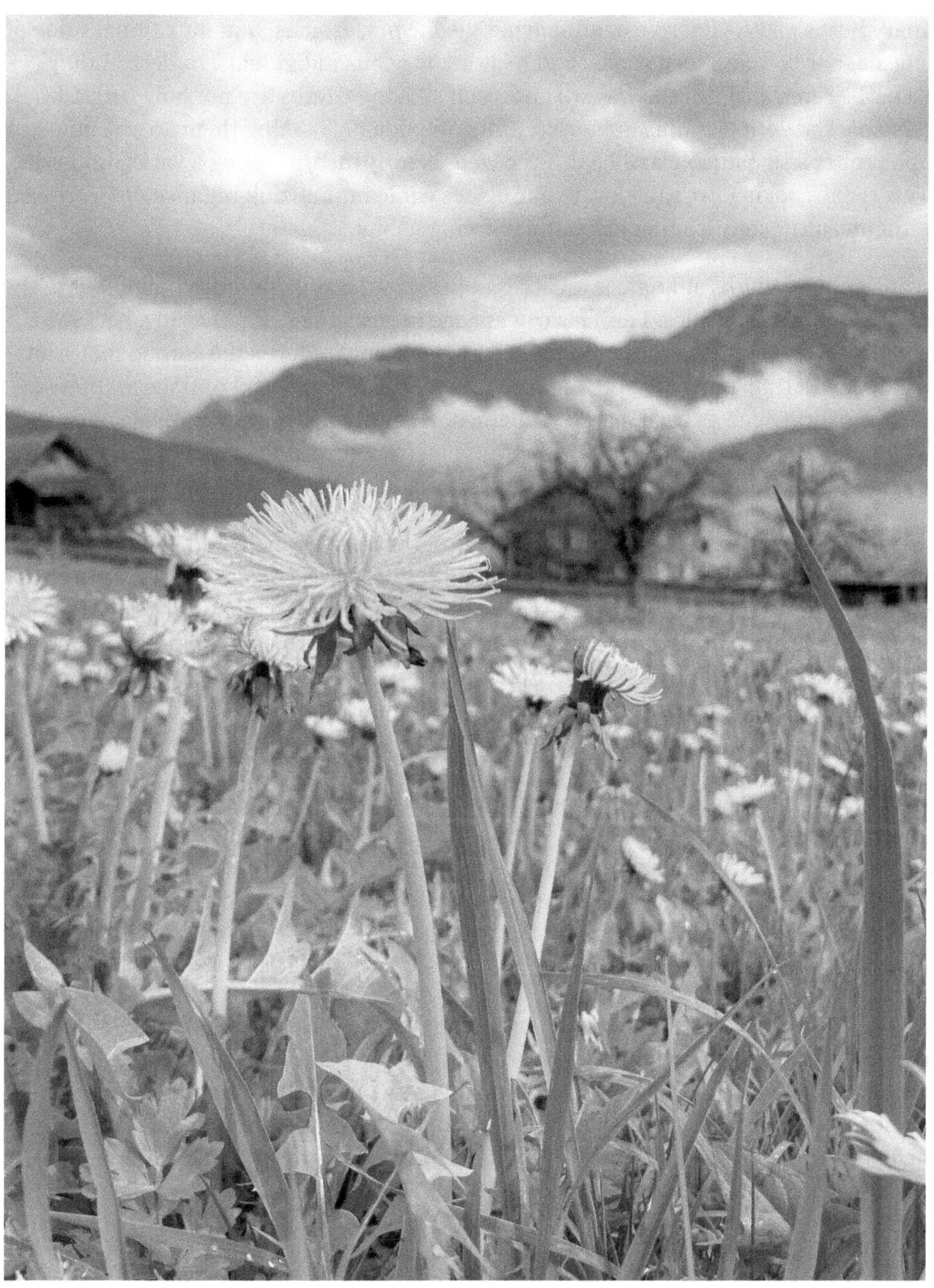

Introduction to Culinary Herbs

Culinary herbs play a vital role in enhancing the flavors, aromas, and nutritional value of our meals. For families, teen cooks, and health-conscious individuals, understanding these herbs can transform the way we approach cooking. Herbs are not only versatile but also packed with vitamins, minerals, and antioxidants, making them an essential component of a sustainable and health-focused diet. By incorporating a variety of herbs into everyday cooking, we can elevate our dishes while minimizing reliance on processed ingredients, ultimately leading to healthier eating habits.

Growing culinary herbs at home is an accessible and rewarding practice that aligns with sustainable living principles. Families can engage in gardening, whether in a backyard, balcony, or even indoors with potted plants. This not only reduces the carbon footprint associated with transporting herbs but also provides fresh, flavorful options at their fingertips. Herbs such as basil, parsley, cilantro, and mint are easy to cultivate and can thrive in various environments, allowing everyone from novice to experienced cooks to enjoy the satisfaction of growing their own ingredients.

In the realm of plant-based meal prep, culinary herbs offer a way to add depth and complexity to dishes without relying on animal products or excessive salt. Fresh herbs can bring vibrancy to vegetable-based recipes, enhancing taste while promoting the use of nutrient-dense superfoods. Incorporating herbs into smoothies, salads, soups, and grain bowls can significantly boost the nutritional profile of meals, ensuring that families and health-conscious cooks receive essential nutrients while enjoying delicious flavors.

Beyond flavor, many culinary herbs possess medicinal properties that can contribute to overall wellness. Herbs like rosemary, thyme, and ginger have been used for centuries not just for their taste but also for their health benefits. They can aid digestion, boost immunity, and even provide anti-inflammatory effects. By integrating these herbs into daily cooking, families can foster a holistic approach to health that emphasizes natural, plant-based solutions to common ailments.

Ultimately, the use of culinary herbs aligns perfectly with low-waste cooking techniques. Herbs can often be used in multiple ways, from fresh garnishes to dried seasonings, ensuring that no part goes to waste. Additionally, utilizing herbs in homemade sauces, dressings, and marinades can reduce the need for store-bought products that typically come in eco-unfriendly packaging. By embracing the versatility of herbs, families can create flavorful meals that are not only good for their health but also beneficial for the planet.

Growing Your Own Herbs at Home

Growing your own herbs at home is an excellent way for families to enhance their culinary experiences while promoting sustainability and health. Herbs are not only easy to grow but also require minimal space and resources, making them ideal for family gardens, balconies, or even kitchen windowsills. By cultivating your own herbs, you can ensure that your family has access to fresh, organic ingredients, reducing reliance on store-bought alternatives that may come packaged in plastic or treated with pesticides.

When starting your herb garden, consider selecting herbs that your family frequently uses in cooking. Basil, parsley, cilantro, and mint are popular choices that thrive in various conditions. These herbs are versatile and can be used in a range of dishes, from salads and sauces to smoothies and teas. Begin by choosing the right containers and soil; drainage is crucial, so opt for pots with holes at the bottom and a high-quality potting mix that retains moisture without becoming waterlogged.

Growing herbs can be an educational and engaging activity for teenagers and younger family members. Encourage them to take part in the planting process, as this hands-on experience fosters a connection to the food they eat. Teach them about the different growth stages of herbs and the importance of sunlight and watering routines. This not only cultivates a sense of responsibility but also promotes an understanding of sustainable food practices, helping to instill a lifelong appreciation for healthy eating.

As your herbs grow, explore creative ways to incorporate them into your family meals. Fresh herbs can elevate the flavor of plant-based dishes, making meals more enjoyable and nutrient-dense. For instance, adding chopped basil to a tomato salad or blending spinach with mint in a smoothie can enhance taste while introducing additional health benefits. By utilizing your homegrown herbs, you can significantly reduce food waste, as fresh herbs can be harvested as needed, minimizing the chances of spoilage.

Lastly, consider the eco-friendly aspects of growing your own herbs. By sourcing seeds or starter plants locally and using organic gardening practices, families can minimize their carbon footprint. Additionally, harvesting herbs from your garden eliminates the need for plastic packaging found in grocery stores. This simple practice not only supports a healthier lifestyle but also contributes to a more sustainable kitchen environment, making it a valuable addition to any family's approach to cooking and meal preparation.

Cooking with Medicinal Ingredients

Cooking with medicinal ingredients is a transformative approach to family meals that not only enhances flavor but also offers a wealth of health benefits. Families can incorporate herbs, spices, and other plant-based ingredients that are known for their medicinal properties into everyday cooking, creating dishes that nourish both the body and the mind. By understanding the unique benefits of these ingredients, home cooks can elevate their culinary practices and foster a deeper connection to the food they prepare.

Herbs such as basil, oregano, and thyme are not only staples in many kitchens but also pack a punch when it comes to health benefits. Basil, for instance, is rich in antioxidants and has anti-inflammatory properties, making it a great addition to sauces, soups, and salads. Oregano is known for its antimicrobial effects and can easily be incorporated into marinades and dressings. By utilizing these herbs fresh or dried, families can enhance the nutritional value of their meals while reducing reliance on processed ingredients that often lack nutritional density.

Spices like turmeric, ginger, and cinnamon are also essential in the realm of medicinal cooking. Turmeric contains curcumin, which has potent anti-inflammatory and antioxidant effects, making it a fantastic addition to curries, rice dishes, and smoothies. Ginger is celebrated for its ability to aid digestion and combat nausea, making it a perfect ingredient for teas and baked goods. Cinnamon not only adds sweetness without sugar but also helps regulate blood sugar levels. These spices can be easily incorporated into various recipes, promoting health while adding warmth and flavor.

In addition to herbs and spices, families can explore the world of superfoods that are locally sourced and nutrient-dense. Ingredients such as kale, beet greens, and quinoa offer significant health benefits and can be found at local farmers' markets or within community-supported agriculture (CSA) programs. These foods can be used in salads, grain bowls, and smoothies, allowing families to create meals that are not only sustainable but also rich in vitamins and minerals. The practice of sourcing ingredients locally supports community farmers and reduces the carbon footprint associated with transporting food.

Finally, incorporating medicinal ingredients into cooking aligns seamlessly with low-waste cooking techniques. By utilizing every part of an ingredient, such as vegetable scraps for broths or herb stems for flavoring, families can minimize waste while maximizing nutrition. Eco-friendly packaging solutions, such as reusable containers for meal prep, further enhance this commitment to sustainability. Combining these practices not only leads to healthier meal options but also encourages a mindful approach to cooking that supports both individual well-being and environmental stewardship.

Chapter 8: Family-Friendly Sustainable Recipes

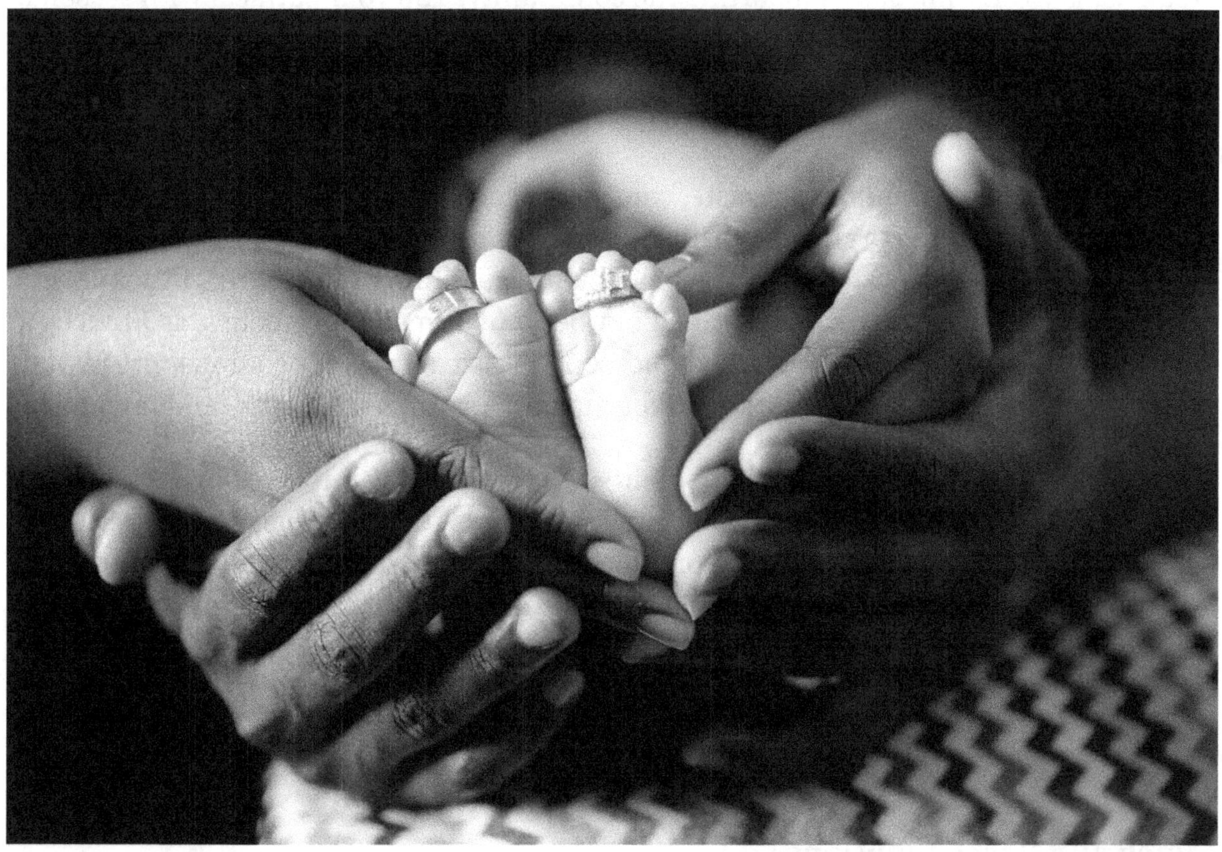

Breakfast Ideas for a Greener Start

Breakfast is often touted as the most important meal of the day, and for good reason. It sets the tone for your energy levels and nutritional intake throughout the morning. For families aiming for a greener start, incorporating sustainable and healthy choices into breakfast can be both fulfilling and enjoyable. This subchapter presents innovative ideas that not only nourish your body but also align with eco-conscious principles, making it easier for families and teen cooks to embrace a more sustainable lifestyle.

One effective way to make your breakfast routine greener is by focusing on plant-based options. Smoothies provide an excellent foundation for nutrient-dense breakfasts. By blending local fruits with leafy greens, such as spinach or kale, you can create a vibrant drink that is rich in vitamins and minerals. To enhance flavor and nutrition, consider adding superfoods like chia seeds, flaxseeds, or even a scoop of local nut butter. These ingredients not only boost the smoothie's health benefits but also reduce dependence on processed products, supporting local farmers and minimizing carbon footprints.

Another fantastic idea for a sustainable breakfast is the use of whole grains. Oatmeal, for instance, is not only inexpensive but can also be customized with a variety of toppings to satisfy different taste preferences. By sourcing oats locally, you can ensure that your breakfast is fresh while also supporting the community. Top your oatmeal with seasonal fruits, nuts, and a drizzle of honey or maple syrup from local producers. This approach reduces packaging waste and encourages a connection to the food source, teaching children the importance of mindful eating.

For families looking to minimize waste, consider incorporating leftovers into breakfast. Utilizing evening meals to create morning dishes can be a fun and resourceful strategy. For example, leftover roasted vegetables can be tossed into scrambled eggs or made into a breakfast hash. Similarly, day-old bread can be transformed into a delicious French toast or a savory strata. This not only reduces food waste but also encourages creativity in the kitchen, allowing young cooks to experiment with different flavors and textures.

Lastly, the packaging of breakfast ingredients can significantly impact your ecological footprint. Choosing bulk bins for grains, nuts, and seeds reduces the use of single-use packaging, while opting for reusable containers for meal prep can streamline your morning routine. Encouraging children and teens to participate in selecting and packing their breakfast ingredients fosters independence and instills lifelong habits of sustainability. By taking small steps to rethink breakfast, families can contribute to a healthier planet while enjoying nourishing meals that set a positive tone for the day ahead.

Lunch and Snack Solutions

Lunch and snack time can often lead to food waste and unhealthy choices, but with a little creativity and planning, families can embrace sustainable and health-conscious solutions. Preparing nutrient-dense meals and snacks not only satisfies hunger but also aligns with a greener lifestyle. By incorporating plant-based ingredients and using locally sourced superfoods, families can craft delicious meals that are both nourishing and environmentally friendly.

One effective strategy for lunch is to create a variety of plant-based wraps and sandwiches. Whole grain tortillas or bread serve as the base for an array of fillings, from hummus and roasted vegetables to avocado and leafy greens. Introducing seasonal produce not only enhances the flavors but also supports local farmers and reduces carbon footprints associated with transport. When planning lunches, consider batch-preparing these wraps at the start of the week, making them readily available for busy days. This method minimizes food waste and ensures that nutritious options are always on hand.

Snacks can often derail a healthy eating plan, but with mindful choices, they can become an opportunity for nourishment. Instead of reaching for processed options, families can prepare homemade snacks using whole, minimally processed ingredients. Energy balls made from oats, nut butter, and dried fruits are an excellent choice. They are easy to make in bulk, can be stored in eco-friendly containers, and provide a quick energy boost that is rich in nutrients. Additionally, incorporating herbal and medicinal foods such as matcha or spirulina into these snacks can enhance their health benefits, making them both functional and delicious.

Smoothies are another versatile option for both lunches and snacks. They allow for the integration of various fruits, vegetables, and superfoods, creating nutrient-dense drinks that can be customized to individual preferences. Families can experiment with different combinations, adding ingredients like spinach, bananas, chia seeds, or local berries. Using reusable containers for smoothie preparation and storage not only cuts down on waste but also encourages families to take their healthy creations on the go. This practice supports hydration and nutrient intake throughout the day.

Finally, implementing low-waste cooking techniques can transform how families approach meal prep and snacks. For instance, utilizing vegetable scraps to make broths or composting organic waste can significantly reduce waste in the kitchen. Encouraging children and teens to participate in these practices fosters a sense of responsibility toward food and the environment. By teaching them to appreciate the full lifecycle of food, families can cultivate a culture of sustainability while enjoying delicious and healthful lunches and snacks that nourish both their bodies and the planet.

Dinner Recipes for All Ages

Dinner recipes that cater to all ages can be both nutritious and exciting, promoting healthy eating habits while minimizing waste. Families often face the challenge of preparing meals that appeal to both children and adults, yet with a little creativity, it is entirely possible to craft dishes that satisfy everyone at the table. By focusing on plant-based ingredients, locally sourced superfoods, and low-waste cooking techniques, families can enjoy delicious dinners that are environmentally friendly and health-conscious.

One versatile dish that can be easily adapted for all ages is a vegetable stir-fry. Utilizing seasonal vegetables from local farmers' markets not only supports the community but also ensures the ingredients are fresh and nutrient-dense. A colorful mix of bell peppers, broccoli, carrots, and snap peas can be quickly sautéed with garlic, ginger, and low-sodium soy sauce or tamari. For added protein, families can include tofu or tempeh, which absorbs flavors wonderfully and can be seasoned to appeal to younger palates. Serving the stir-fry over whole grains like brown rice or quinoa creates a well-rounded meal, while any leftovers can be repurposed into a nutritious lunch the next day.

Another delightful option is a build-your-own taco night, which encourages creativity and self-expression at the dinner table. Begin with a base of soft corn tortillas or lettuce wraps, which are low-waste and gluten-free alternatives. Provide a variety of fillings such as seasoned black beans, roasted sweet potatoes, and sautéed mushrooms. Toppings can include avocado, salsa, shredded lettuce, and fresh herbs, allowing each family member to customize their meal according to their taste preferences. This not only makes dinner more engaging but also introduces children to the concept of balanced meals and the importance of incorporating diverse flavors.

For families interested in smoothies, a nutrient-dense smoothie bowl serves as a playful and nutritious dinner alternative. By blending frozen fruits like bananas, berries, and spinach with a splash of plant-based milk, families can create a thick, creamy base. Toppings such as granola, nuts, seeds, and fresh fruit add texture and visual appeal. This dish is not only quick to prepare but can also be a fun way to involve teens in the kitchen, encouraging them to experiment with flavors and ingredients while utilizing leftover fruits and veggies that might otherwise go to waste.

Finally, consider incorporating herbal and medicinal foods into dinner recipes as a way to boost health benefits. A simple herbal pesto made from fresh basil, garlic, nuts, and a splash of olive oil can elevate pasta dishes or roasted vegetables, providing a flavorful punch while promoting wellness. Families can engage children in the cooking process by teaching them about the health benefits of different herbs and how to grow their own at home, fostering a deeper connection to their food. By utilizing these strategies, families can create dinners that are not only appealing to all ages but also align with sustainable cooking practices and a commitment to reducing waste.

Chapter 9: Engaging Teen Cooks in Sustainable Practices

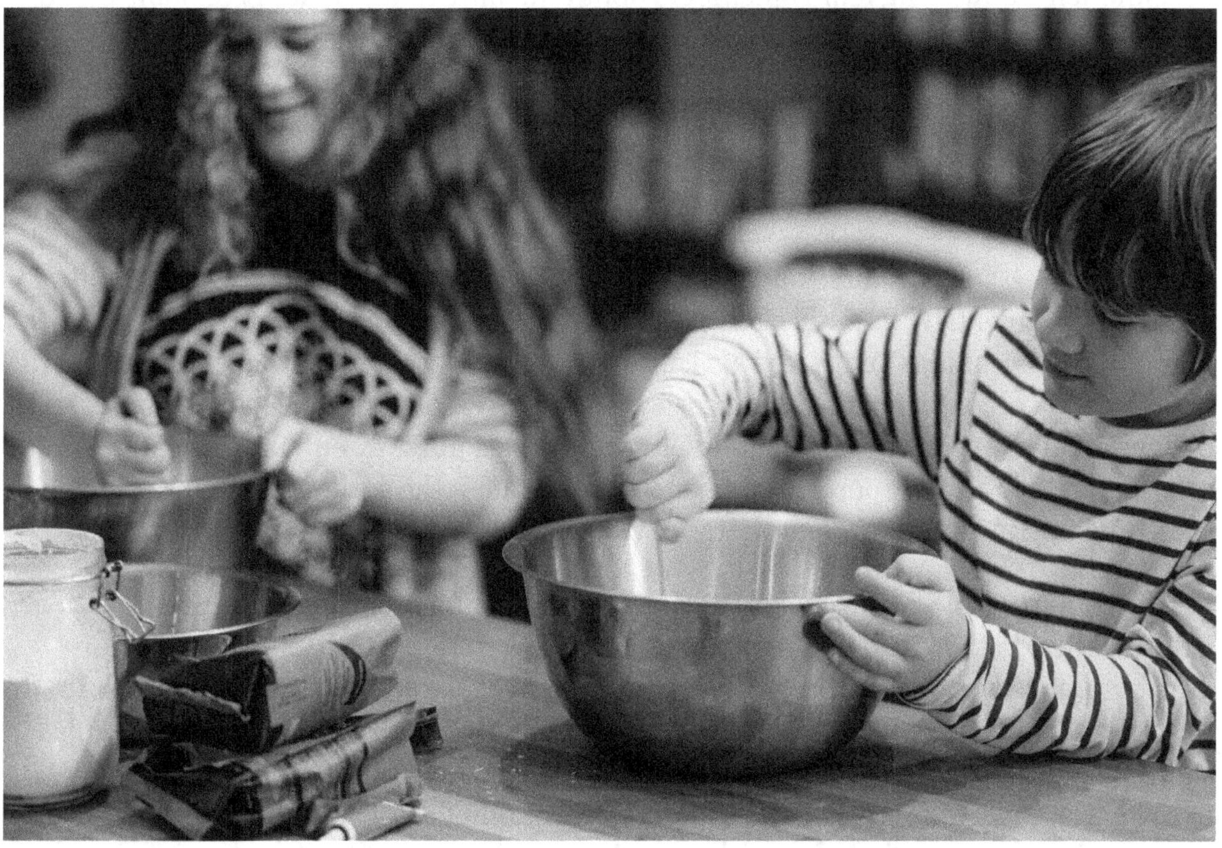

Teaching Kitchen Skills

Teaching kitchen skills is an essential step toward fostering a sustainable and health-conscious cooking environment in your home. By equipping family members, especially teen cooks, with practical kitchen skills, you empower them to create nutritious meals while minimizing waste. These skills not only enhance culinary confidence but also encourage a deeper understanding of the ingredients chosen for each dish. As families embrace the principles of sustainable cooking, the kitchen becomes a space for creativity, experimentation, and learning.

One of the foundational skills to teach is the proper handling and preparation of fresh produce. Families should learn how to wash, peel, and chop fruits and vegetables efficiently, focusing on techniques that reduce waste. For example, using a vegetable peeler instead of a knife can help retain more of the edible skin, which is often rich in nutrients. Additionally, families can explore different ways to utilize vegetable scraps, such as making homemade stocks or composting, thereby contributing to a more sustainable kitchen ecosystem.

Incorporating plant-based meal prep into family routines is another key area for skill development. Educating family members about the nutritional benefits of plant-based ingredients can inspire them to create dishes that are both delicious and healthful. Teaching techniques such as batch cooking, which involves preparing large quantities of meals for the week ahead, can save time and reduce food waste. By learning to store and freeze leftovers properly, families can ensure that no food goes to waste while enjoying the convenience of ready-to-eat meals.

Understanding how to source and select locally grown superfoods empowers families to make environmentally friendly choices. Teaching cooks how to navigate local farmers' markets or community-supported agriculture programs can deepen their connection to the food they prepare. Families can learn to identify seasonal produce, which tends to be fresher, tastier, and more sustainable. This knowledge not only enhances meal preparation but also supports local farmers and reduces the carbon footprint associated with transporting food over long distances.

Lastly, exploring low-waste cooking techniques is vital for fostering a culture of sustainability in the kitchen. Families can learn how to repurpose leftovers, create nutrient-dense smoothies from overripe fruits and vegetables, and utilize herbs for both flavor and health benefits. Encouraging experimentation with eco-friendly packaging solutions, like reusable containers and wraps, can also help reduce reliance on single-use plastics. By instilling these skills and values, families can transform their cooking practices into a more mindful, health-conscious, and sustainable lifestyle.

Involving Teens in Meal Planning

Involving teens in meal planning can significantly enhance their cooking skills while fostering a sense of responsibility and awareness about food choices. As families strive to adopt more sustainable practices, engaging teens in this process not only empowers them but also cultivates a deeper understanding of nutrition and environmental impact. By including teens in meal planning, families can create a dynamic cooking environment where everyone contributes ideas and preferences, leading to more enjoyable and nutritious meals.

To begin, consider hosting a family meal planning session where everyone can share their favorite dishes and explore new recipes together. This collaborative approach encourages teens to think critically about the ingredients they choose and how those ingredients align with healthful eating. Highlighting the benefits of plant-based options and locally sourced superfoods can inspire them to experiment with different flavors and textures. This is an excellent opportunity to educate them on the nutritional value of various foods and how to balance meals effectively.

Another effective strategy is to assign specific roles to teens during the meal planning process. For example, one teen could focus on researching seasonal produce available at local farmers' markets, while another could be tasked with finding recipes that utilize these ingredients. By giving them responsibilities, parents instill a sense of ownership over the meals they create. This hands-on experience not only builds their confidence in the kitchen but also reinforces the importance of supporting local food systems and reducing the carbon footprint associated with food transportation.

Incorporating eco-friendly packaging solutions into the meal planning process is another way to engage teens in sustainability. Discussing the impact of single-use plastics and encouraging the use of reusable containers can help them understand the broader implications of their choices. When planning lunches or snacks, involve teens in selecting packaging that minimizes waste, such as beeswax wraps or glass containers. This practice not only reduces waste but also empowers them to make environmentally conscious decisions in their everyday lives.

Finally, introducing nutrient-dense smoothies into the meal planning routine can be an enjoyable way to involve teens in healthy eating. Encourage them to experiment with various fruits, vegetables, and superfoods, allowing them to create their own unique recipes. This not only promotes creativity in the kitchen but also highlights the importance of incorporating a variety of nutrients into their diets. By making meal planning a fun and interactive experience, families can instill lifelong habits of health-conscious cooking and sustainable living in their teens.

Creating a Family Cooking Challenge

Creating a family cooking challenge is a wonderful way to engage everyone in the kitchen while fostering creativity and promoting sustainability. This interactive experience allows family members to experiment with various ingredients, particularly those that are plant-based and locally sourced. By establishing a friendly competition, families can explore new cooking techniques, reduce waste, and enhance their culinary skills together. The challenge can also serve as an opportunity to educate younger family members about the importance of nutrition and the environmental impact of food choices.

To kick off the family cooking challenge, set clear themes or goals that align with your family's health-conscious values. For instance, you could focus on plant-based meal prep, where each family member is tasked with creating a dish using seasonal vegetables and fruits sourced from local farmers' markets. This not only encourages creativity but also fosters a sense of community by supporting local agriculture. Each week, the family can vote on their favorite dish, creating a fun and competitive spirit while also learning about the benefits of eating fresh, local produce.

Incorporating low-waste cooking techniques into the challenge can further enhance the experience. Encourage family members to think critically about how to utilize every part of an ingredient. For instance, vegetable scraps can be saved to make broths, while overripe fruits can be transformed into smoothies or baked goods. Providing guidelines for eco-friendly packaging solutions can also be part of the challenge, prompting participants to bring their own containers for leftovers or to find ways to eliminate single-use plastics in their cooking processes.

Another engaging aspect of the cooking challenge can be the inclusion of nutrient-dense smoothie recipes. Designate a day where family members create their own smoothie concoctions, focusing on incorporating superfoods and herbal ingredients that offer health benefits. This not only makes for a delicious treat but also educates everyone on the value of incorporating various nutrients into their diets. You can even introduce a "smoothie of the week" that highlights different seasonal fruits and vegetables, making it a fun and educational experience.

Finally, documenting the cooking challenge can provide a sense of accomplishment and serve as a valuable resource for future meals. Encourage family members to take photos of their dishes, write down their recipes, and share their experiences. This not only strengthens family bonds but also creates a collection of sustainable and health-conscious recipes that can be revisited and refined over time. The family cooking challenge can evolve into a cherished tradition that nurtures creativity, reinforces healthy eating habits, and fosters a commitment to sustainability in the kitchen.

Chapter 10: Building a Sustainable Kitchen Culture

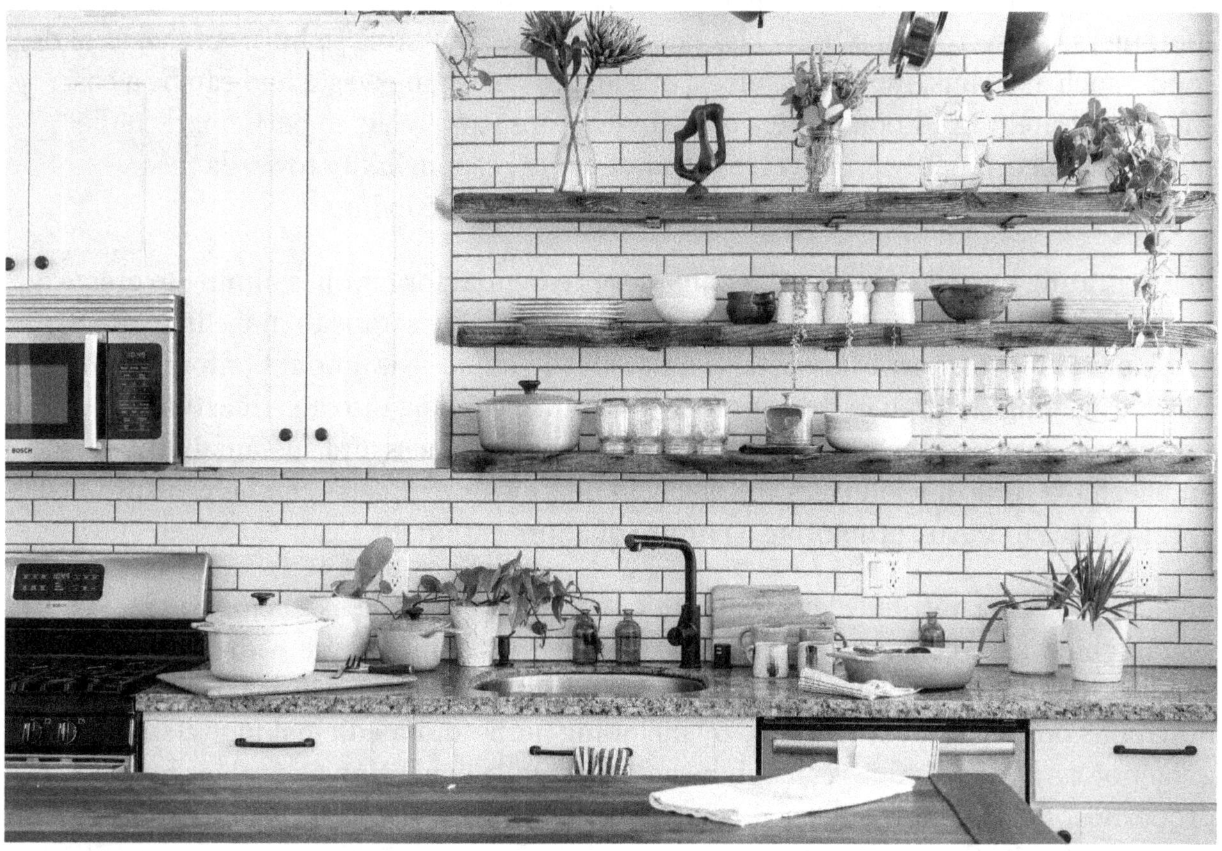

Creating Sustainable Kitchen Routines

Creating sustainable kitchen routines is essential for families eager to minimize their environmental impact while promoting health and wellness. A sustainable kitchen begins with mindful shopping practices, prioritizing locally sourced ingredients and seasonal produce. By opting for fresh, organic fruits and vegetables from local farmers' markets or community-supported agriculture (CSA) programs, families not only support their local economy but also reduce the carbon footprint associated with long-distance food transport. This practice encourages the consumption of nutrient-dense foods that are at their peak flavor and nutritional value, contributing to a healthier diet.

Meal planning is a cornerstone of sustainable kitchen routines. By organizing weekly meals in advance, families can make efficient use of ingredients, preventing food waste and ensuring that everything purchased is utilized. This approach allows for creative meal prep, emphasizing plant-based recipes that incorporate a variety of superfoods like quinoa, lentils, and leafy greens. When planning meals, consider batch cooking to create versatile dishes that can be repurposed throughout the week, such as using roasted vegetables in salads, grain bowls, or as toppings for whole-grain pizzas. This not only saves time but also fosters an environment of resourcefulness in the kitchen.

Eco-friendly packaging solutions are another vital aspect of sustainable kitchen routines. Families can significantly reduce plastic waste by opting for reusable containers, beeswax wraps, and glass jars for storage. Investing in bulk purchases of dry goods, such as grains, nuts, and spices, minimizes packaging waste and can be a cost-effective strategy. Additionally, encouraging children and teens to participate in the selection of eco-friendly products fosters a sense of responsibility towards the environment and teaches valuable life skills in sustainable living.

Incorporating low-waste cooking techniques is essential for families aiming to create a greener kitchen. Simple practices, such as using vegetable scraps to make homemade broth or composting organic waste, can drastically reduce the amount of food thrown away. Engaging children in these practices can turn cooking into an educational experience, teaching them the importance of resourcefulness and sustainability. Furthermore, utilizing leftovers creatively in new meals or snacks can help ensure that nothing goes to waste, promoting a culture of appreciation for food.

Finally, exploring nutrient-dense smoothie recipes can provide a delicious and sustainable way to consume fruits and vegetables. Smoothies made with seasonal produce, combined with superfoods like chia seeds or spirulina, offer an easy and nutritious option for busy families. By including herbs and medicinal foods, such as ginger or turmeric, families can enhance flavors while benefiting from their health properties. This not only aligns with sustainable practices but also encourages health-conscious habits that can be enjoyed by the whole family, fostering a love for nutritious food and a commitment to sustainable living.

Encouraging Eco-Friendly Habits

Encouraging eco-friendly habits in the kitchen is essential for families aiming to create a sustainable living environment. With the increasing awareness of environmental issues, adopting practices that minimize waste and promote sustainability can significantly impact our planet. Simple changes in cooking techniques and food preparation can lead to healthier meals and reduce the overall carbon footprint. By integrating eco-friendly habits into daily routines, families can create a culture of sustainability that benefits both their health and the environment.

One of the most effective ways to encourage eco-friendly habits is through plant-based meal preparation. By incorporating more plant-based meals into the family diet, not only can families improve their health by consuming nutrient-dense foods, but they can also lessen the demand for meat production, which is known to be resource-intensive. Planning meals around seasonal vegetables and legumes not only enhances the nutritional profile but also encourages the use of locally sourced ingredients, thereby supporting local farmers and reducing transportation-related emissions.

An essential aspect of eco-friendly cooking is understanding food waste and finding ways to minimize it. Families can adopt low-waste cooking techniques, such as utilizing vegetable scraps to make broths or composting leftover food. By being mindful of portion sizes and creatively repurposing leftovers, families can significantly reduce their kitchen waste. This not only teaches valuable lessons about resourcefulness but also instills a sense of responsibility towards food consumption and waste management.

In addition to meal prep, using eco-friendly packaging solutions is another key component of sustainable cooking. Families can invest in reusable containers, beeswax wraps, and biodegradable bags to reduce single-use plastics in the kitchen. Encouraging children and teens to participate in choosing sustainable packaging can foster a sense of ownership and commitment to eco-friendly practices. Additionally, when shopping for ingredients, opting for products with minimal or no packaging not only supports sustainability but also often leads to healthier choices.

Finally, creating a habit of making nutrient-dense smoothies can be a fun and engaging way for families to incorporate superfoods into their diets. By blending a variety of fruits, vegetables, and herbs, families can experiment with flavors while maximizing health benefits. Smoothies also serve as an excellent opportunity to use up overripe fruits or leftover greens, minimizing waste. Encouraging teens to take the lead in smoothie preparation can empower them to explore healthy eating habits and develop a lifelong commitment to sustainability in the kitchen. By fostering these eco-friendly practices, families can contribute to a healthier planet while enjoying delicious and nutritious meals together.

Celebrating Successes Together

Celebrating successes together in the kitchen not only fosters a sense of community but also reinforces the values of sustainability and health-conscious cooking that are essential for a greener family kitchen. When families come together to prepare meals, share recipes, or even embark on new cooking techniques, they create an environment that encourages collaboration and creativity. This shared experience not only enhances the cooking process but also strengthens family bonds, making healthy eating a collective goal rather than an individual task.

One effective way to celebrate culinary achievements is by organizing themed cooking nights. Families can choose specific themes based on seasonal ingredients or cultural cuisines that promote the use of locally sourced superfoods. For example, a Mediterranean night could incorporate fresh vegetables, legumes, and herbs, allowing each family member to contribute a dish. This approach not only diversifies the menu but also provides an opportunity to educate everyone about the nutritional benefits of various ingredients while enjoying the process of cooking together.

Another rewarding practice is to document and share the successes achieved in the kitchen. Families can create a shared recipe book or an online blog where they post their favorite plant-based meal prep ideas, low-waste cooking techniques, and nutrient-dense smoothie recipes. This not only serves as a personal archive of culinary adventures but also allows families to inspire others in their community to adopt similar practices. By sharing successes, families can cultivate a network of support and motivation, making healthy cooking a more enjoyable journey.

Celebrating milestones, such as completing a week of zero-waste meals or trying a new cooking technique, can also be an uplifting experience. Families can host small gatherings or potlucks where they showcase their dishes, emphasizing the eco-friendly packaging solutions they employed or the herbal and medicinal foods they incorporated. Recognizing these achievements, whether big or small, reinforces the importance of sustainable cooking practices and encourages everyone to continue exploring new culinary horizons.

Lastly, engaging in community events focused on sustainable cooking can be a powerful way to celebrate collective achievements. Participating in local farmers' markets, cooking workshops, or sustainability fairs allows families to connect with like-minded individuals who share their passion for health-conscious cooking. These interactions not only enhance their knowledge but also provide a platform for sharing experiences and successes. By celebrating together, families can inspire and be inspired, creating a ripple effect that promotes a healthier, more sustainable way of living.

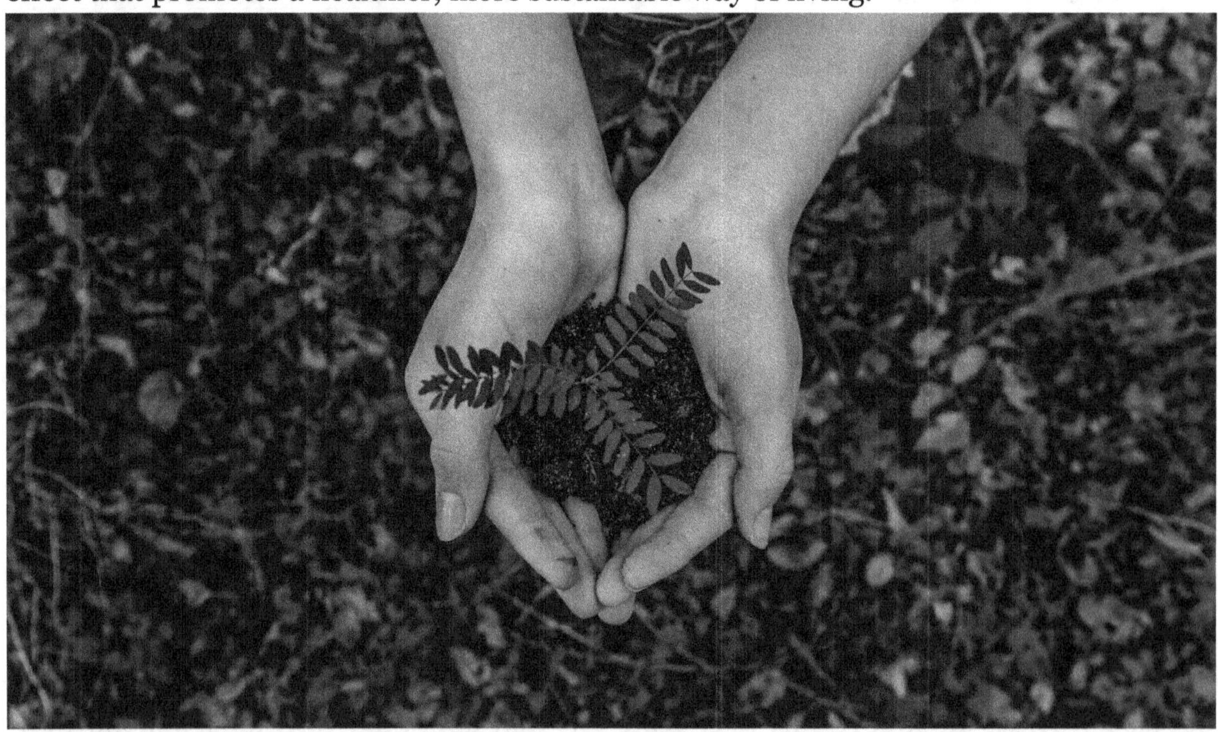

RECIPIES:

Here are a few sustainable family recipes to include in your familys' journey

<u>1. Root-to-Stem Veggie Stir-Fry</u>

This colorful stir-fry makes use of the entire vegetable, from root to stem, reducing waste and maximizing nutrition.

Ingredients:

- 1 cup broccoli stems, peeled and thinly sliced
- 2 cups broccoli florets
- 1 large carrot, thinly sliced (use carrot tops for garnish)
- 1 bunch of Swiss chard, stems chopped and leaves sliced
- 1 bell pepper, sliced
- 2 garlic cloves, minced
- 2 tbsp soy sauce or tamari
- 1 tbsp sesame oil
- 1 tbsp olive oil
- 1 tsp grated ginger
- Cooked rice or quinoa, for serving

Instructions:

1. Heat olive oil in a large pan over medium heat. Add the garlic and ginger, and sauté for 1-2 minutes.
2. Add the broccoli stems and Swiss chard stems to the pan, cooking for 3-4 minutes until they start to soften.
3. Add the broccoli florets, bell pepper, and carrot slices, and stir-fry for another 3-5 minutes.
4. Add the soy sauce and sesame oil, stirring well to combine. Cook until all vegetables are tender but still crisp.
5. Serve over cooked rice or quinoa, and garnish with carrot tops for a fresh, herbaceous finish.

<u>2. Leftover Lentil Shepherd's Pie</u>

Turn leftover cooked lentils and mashed potatoes into a hearty family meal with this plant-based take on a classic comfort dish.

Ingredients:

* 2 cups cooked lentils
* 1 onion, diced
* 2 garlic cloves, minced
* 1 carrot, diced
* 1 celery stalk, diced
* 1 cup vegetable broth
* 1 tbsp tomato paste
* 2 tsp thyme
* 2 cups leftover mashed potatoes
* 1 tbsp olive oil
* Salt and pepper, to taste

Instructions:

1. Preheat oven to 375°F (190°C).
2. Heat olive oil in a large skillet over medium heat. Add onion, garlic, carrot, and celery, and cook until softened, about 5 minutes.
3. Stir in the cooked lentils, tomato paste, thyme, and vegetable broth. Simmer for 10 minutes until the mixture thickens slightly. Season with salt and pepper.
4. Transfer the lentil mixture to a baking dish. Spread the leftover mashed potatoes evenly over the top.
5. Bake for 20-25 minutes, until the top is golden and crispy. Serve hot.

3. Zero-Waste Vegetable Broth

Use kitchen scraps to create a flavorful broth that can be used as a base for soups, stews, or cooking grains.

Ingredients:

* 2 cups vegetable scraps (carrot peels, onion skins, garlic ends, celery tops, herb stems, etc.)
* 8 cups water
* 2 bay leaves
* 1 tsp peppercorns
* 1 tsp salt
* 1 tbsp olive oil (optional)

Instructions:

1.   Place vegetable scraps in a large pot and cover with water. Add bay leaves, peppercorns, and salt.

2.   Bring to a boil, then reduce heat and simmer for 45 minutes to an hour.

3.   Strain the broth through a fine-mesh sieve, discarding the solids. If desired, add olive oil for a richer broth.

4.   Store in airtight containers in the refrigerator for up to 5 days, or freeze for later use.

4. Carrot Top Pesto

Don't toss those carrot tops! Use them to make a delicious, waste-free pesto that pairs well with pasta, roasted vegetables, or sandwiches.

Ingredients:

- 1 cup carrot tops (leaves only, washed and dried)
- 1 cup fresh basil leaves
- 1/3 cup olive oil
- 1/4 cup sunflower seeds or pumpkin seeds
- 2 garlic cloves
- 1 tbsp lemon juice
- Salt and pepper, to taste

Instructions:

1.   In a food processor, combine carrot tops, basil, garlic, and seeds. Pulse until coarsely chopped.

2.   Slowly stream in olive oil while processing until smooth.

3.   Add lemon juice, salt, and pepper to taste, and pulse to combine.

4.   Store in a jar in the refrigerator for up to a week. Use as a sauce for pasta, a spread for sandwiches, or a dip for veggies.

5. Day-Old Bread Frittata

Turn stale bread into a delicious frittata packed with veggies and protein. This is a great way to use up leftover vegetables and bread.

Ingredients:

- 4 slices of stale bread, torn into pieces

- 6 eggs
- 1/2 cup milk or plant-based milk
- 1 cup cooked or raw vegetables (leftover roasted veggies, spinach, etc.)
- 1/2 cup shredded cheese (optional)
- 1 tsp olive oil
- Salt and pepper, to taste

Instructions:

1. Preheat the oven to 350°F (175°C).
2. In a large bowl, whisk together eggs, milk, salt, and pepper. Add torn bread and let it soak for a few minutes.
3. Stir in the vegetables and cheese, if using.
4. Heat olive oil in an oven-safe skillet over medium heat. Pour in the egg mixture and cook for 3-4 minutes, until the edges begin to set.
5. Transfer the skillet to the oven and bake for 15-20 minutes, until the frittata is fully cooked and golden on top. Serve warm.

These recipes showcase how easy it can be to embrace sustainable practices in the kitchen while creating delicious family meals.

REFERENCES:

Here are some excellent resources for further reading on sustainable cooking and reducing kitchen waste:

1. "Waste Not: How to Get the Most from Your Food" by James Beard Foundation
- This book is a comprehensive guide that provides tips and recipes for using up every part of the ingredients you buy. It emphasizes reducing waste in the kitchen and highlights various ways to repurpose food scraps creatively.
2. "The Everlasting Meal: Cooking with Economy and Grace" by Tamar Adler
- Adler's book is a philosophical take on how to cook more sustainably and thoughtfully, focusing on making the most of what you have. It's filled with practical advice on cooking with economy and making meals from scratch using simple ingredients.
3. "The Zero-Waste Chef: Plant-Forward Recipes and Tips for a Sustainable Kitchen and Planet" by Anne-Marie Bonneau
- This cookbook is specifically tailored for those looking to reduce waste in their cooking habits. It offers plant-based, low-waste recipes and strategies for organizing your kitchen in a more sustainable way.

4.   "Cooking with Scraps: Turn Your Peels, Cores, Rinds, and Stems into Delicious Meals" by Lindsay-Jean Hard
   • This book is full of inventive recipes for using ingredients that most people throw away. It provides great inspiration for reducing waste and making the most of every ingredient, from vegetable peel chips to fruit scrap-infused syrups.
5.   "The Waste-Free Kitchen Handbook: A Guide to Eating Well and Saving Money by Wasting Less Food" by Dana Gunders
   • Gunders' handbook is a concise guide to reducing food waste, with practical tips on planning meals, storing food properly, and repurposing leftovers.
6.   "Root to Leaf: A Southern Chef Cooks Through the Seasons" by Steven Satterfield
   • While not exclusively about waste reduction, this book emphasizes seasonal, plant-based cooking and provides ideas for using every part of a vegetable, reflecting the root-to-stem philosophy.
7.   "Nose to Tail Eating: A Kind of British Cooking" by Fergus Henderson
   • Henderson's philosophy centers around using the entire animal, which aligns with waste-reduction principles in cooking. While this book is more focused on meat, it's a good resource for those looking to adopt sustainable practices in animal-based cooking.
8.   "Sustainable Kitchen: Recipes and Inspiration for Plant-Based, Planet-Conscious Meals" by Heather Wolfe and Jaynie McCloskey
   • This cookbook offers plant-based recipes that emphasize sustainability, along with tips on reducing waste, sourcing eco-friendly ingredients, and mindful cooking.
9.   "Animal, Vegetable, Miracle: A Year of Food Life" by Barbara Kingsolver
   • This memoir chronicles the author's year of living and eating sustainably, focusing on local, seasonal foods. While it's not a recipe book, it offers inspiration for a sustainable lifestyle and eco-friendly eating habits.
10.   "The Art of Fermentation" by Sandor Ellix Katz

   • This book dives deep into fermentation as a method for preserving food and extending its usefulness, a key technique in sustainable cooking. It's a great resource for anyone interested in reducing waste through fermentation.

These books and resources provide a solid foundation for learning more about sustainable cooking and how to minimize waste in the kitchen. They offer both philosophical perspectives and practical tips for making eco-conscious choices.

Dear Reader,

Thank you so much for joining me on this journey through Waste Knot: Creative Cooking Techniques for a Greener Family Kitchen. I am deeply grateful that you've chosen to spend time with this book, and I hope it has inspired you to think differently about your kitchen, your meals, and the small steps you can take toward a more sustainable lifestyle.

Every effort you make, whether it's repurposing leftovers, choosing to compost, or finding creative uses for food scraps, brings us one step closer to living in harmony with our planet. It's easy to feel overwhelmed by the scale of environmental challenges, but I truly believe that change begins at home, with the choices we make every day. The kitchen, the heart of the home, is one of the best places to start.

As you apply the techniques and recipes from this book, remember that sustainability isn't about perfection—it's about progress. Every time you take a step toward reducing waste or choosing more eco-friendly options, you are making a difference. These small actions, when taken together, add up to a larger impact that benefits not just our families, but future generations.

I want to encourage you to keep experimenting, keep learning, and keep sharing your knowledge with those around you. Together, we can create a ripple effect that extends far beyond our own homes, influencing our communities and the world at large. Living sustainably is an ongoing journey, one that invites creativity, flexibility, and even fun!

Thank you again for allowing me to be a part of your sustainable cooking adventure. I'm excited to see what you create, how you grow, and the changes you inspire along the way.

With gratitude and encouragement,

Monica Lynne Chase

FIN